www.bma.org.uk/library

KT-472-672

Get Through
MRCPsych: MCQs for Paper I

Arunraj Kaimal MBBS MRCPsych
Consultant Old Age Psychiatrist and Honorary Lecturer in Psychiatry,
Wythenshawe Hospital, Manchester, UK

Manoj Rajagopal MBBS MRCPsych MSc
ST-5 in Old Age Psychiatry, Hope Hospital, Manchester, UK

Salman Karim MBBS FCPS MSc
Consultant Old Age Psychiatrist and Honorary Lecturer in Psychiatry,
Hope Hospital, Manchester, UK

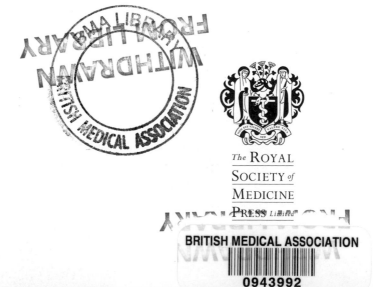

The ROYAL
SOCIETY of
MEDICINE
PRESS Limited

WITHDRAWN FROM BMA LIBRARY
BRITISH MEDICAL ASSOCIATION

BRITISH MEDICAL ASSOCIATION
0943992

© 2009 Royal Society of Medicine Press Ltd

Published by the Royal Society of Medicine Press Ltd
1 Wimpole Street, London W1G 0AE, UK
Tel: +44 (0)20 7290 2921
Fax: +44 (0)20 7290 2929
E-mail: publishing@rsm.ac.uk
Website: www.rsmpress.co.uk

Apart from any fair dealing for the purposes of research or private study, criticism or review, as permitted under the UK Copyright, Designs and Patents Act, 1988, no part of this publication may be reproduced, stored or transmitted, in any form or by any means, without the prior permission in writing of the publishers or in the case of reprographic reproduction in accordance with the terms of licences issued by the Copyright Licensing Agency in the UK, or in accordance with the terms of licences issued by the appropriate Reproduction Rights Organization outside the UK. Enquiries concerning reproduction outside the terms stated here should be sent to the publishers at the UK address printed on this page.

The rights of Arunraj Kaimal, Manoj Rajagopal and Salman Karim to be identified as authors of this work have been asserted by them in accordance with the Copyright, Designs and Patents Act, 1988.

British Library Cataloguing in Publication Data
A catalogue record for this book is available from the British Library

ISBN: 978-1-85315-843-8

Distribution in Europe and Rest of World:
Marston Book Services Ltd
PO Box 269
Abingdon
Oxon OX14 4YN, UK
Tel: +44 (0)1235 465500
Fax: +44 (0)1235 465555
Email: direct.order@marston.co.uk

Distribution in the USA and Canada:
Royal Society of Medicine Press Ltd
c/o BookMasters Inc
30 Amberwood Parkway
Ashland, OH 44805, USA
Tel: +1 800 247 6553/+1 800 266 5564
Fax: +1 419 281 6883
Email: order@bookmasters.com

Distribution in Australia and New Zealand:
Elsevier Australia
30–52 Smidmore Street
Marrickville NSW 2204, Australia
Tel: +61 2 9517 8999
Fax: +61 2 9517 2249
Email: service@elsevier.com.au

Typeset by Techset Composition Limited, Salisbury, UK
Printed and bound in Great Britain by Bell & Bain, Glasgow

Contents

Introduction

The examination

The new MRCPsych exam consists of three written papers and one clinical exam (the CASC). There have been major changes to the exam's format recently, the most important being the change from individual statement questions (ISQs) and extended matching items (EMIs) to 'best answer 1 of 5' style multiple choice questions (MCQs) and EMIs. Although there are a number of ISQ and EMI books available on the market, there are very few dedicated solely to the new-format 'best answer 1 of 5' MCQs.

In this book we have attempted to overcome this shortfall by providing 640 MCQs covering all areas of the MRCPsych Paper 1 curriculum. The presentation of questions in this book according to the subheadings in the new curriculum will make revision easier, making this book an essential companion for trainees preparing for the MRCPsych Paper 1 exam.

As described in the curriculum, each MCQ comprises a question stem, which is usually one or two sentences long but may be longer. The question stem is followed by a list of five options; candidates should choose the single option that best fits the question stem.

The MRCPsych Paper 1 exam is 3 hours long and contains 200 questions. Approximately one-third of the exam will be the EMI component. Candidates are advised to attempt all questions. No marks are deducted for incorrect answers. One mark is given for the correct answer.

Revising for the examination

One key to success is to practise MCQs in the subject areas that regularly appear in the exam. We have covered all such areas in this book and provided a list of books useful in revision as well as the essential reference textbooks. We have used these books for reference in writing this MCQ book.

The best way to practise MCQs is in groups of candidates preparing for the exam. In small groups, the recommended practice method is to solve MCQs by reading around the topic, and then compare the answers and explanations given in the book. It is important to remember that this book is not a substitute for standard textbooks and should be used as a guide to focus on important exam topics. In this book we have not included page numbers of textbooks within the answers. Candidates are expected to read around the topics covered in the MCQ stem from the further reading references detailed at the end of the answer section in each chapter.

In the later part of revision, that is a few weeks before the exam, this book should be used as a practice exam, and 10 questions from each chapter should be solved in 2 hours (altogether 120 questions in one sitting), since the actual examination is 3 hours long and two-thirds of it consists of MCQs. Choosing different sets of multiples of 10 each time (for example, question numbers 1–10 from each chapter for the first practice examination and 11–20 for the second) will give the trainee the opportunity to undertake at least five practice exams before going into the actual exam. Good time management is an important contributor to success and strict time keeping is essential in preparation for the exam.

It is also important to read and understand each stem thoroughly since some common terms used in MCQs may guide you to the correct response. Although there is no strict rule that a given term can indicate whether the statement is true or false, the use of terms such as 'may', 'may be', 'can occur', 'can be', etc, could indicate an increased chance of the statement being true. Similarly, terms such as 'always occur' and 'never occur' could indicate the possibility of the statement being false.

Other terms such as 'characteristic', 'pathognomonic', 'common' and 'rare' should also be interpreted cautiously. Generally, 'characteristic' means that without the presence of that feature you doubt the diagnosis; a 'pathognomonic' feature is found only in that condition; 'common' generally means found in more than 30%; and 'rare' means found in less than 5%.

We recommend working through the chapters of this book as early as possible before the exam date, reading around the topics given in a question stem from the books provided in the reading list and making notes for reference a few weeks before the exam. We suggest that you attempt the questions before checking the answers and any questions answered incorrectly should be noted and revised carefully in the weeks just before the exam. In this way we hope this book will be useful for consolidating your knowledge and helping you to get through the MRCPsych Paper 1 exam.

Arunraj Kaimal
Manoj Rajagopal
Salman Karim

Recommended reading

Preparation for the Paper 1 exam

British National Formulary. *BNF 57*. London: Pharmaceutical Press. Also available at: www.bnf.org/bnf.

Buckley P, Prewette D, Bird J, Harrison G. *Examination Notes in Psychiatry*, 4th edn. London: Hodder Education, 2004.

Gelder M, Harrison P, Cowen P. *Shorter Oxford Textbook of Psychiatry*, 5th edn. Oxford: Oxford University Press, 2006.

Hodges JR. *Cognitive Assessment for Clinicians*, 2nd edn. Oxford: Oxford University Press, 2007.

ICD-10: *The ICD-10 Classification of Mental and Behavioural Disorders: Clinical Descriptions and Diagnostic Guidelines*. Geneva: World Health Organization, 1990.

Munafo M. *Psychology for the MRCPsych*, 2nd edn. London: Hodder Education, 2002.

Oyebode F. *Sims' Symptoms in the Mind: An Introduction to Descriptive Psychopathology*, 4th edn. London: Saunders, 2008.

Puri B, Hall A. *Revision Notes in Psychiatry*, 2nd edn. London: Arnold/ Hodder Education, 2004.

Sadock BJ, Sadock VA. *Kaplan and Sadock's Synopsis of Psychiatry*, 10th edn. Baltimore, MD: Lippincott Williams and Wilkins, 2008.

Smith EE, Bem DJ, Nolen-Hoeksema S. Chapters 2–6. In: *Atkinson and Hilgard's Introduction to Psychology*, 14th edn. Florence, KY: Wadsworth Publishing Company, 2003.

Taylor D, Paton C, Robert Kerwin R. *Maudsley Prescribing Guidelines*, 9th edn. London: Informa Healthcare, 2007.

Wright P, Stern J, Phelan M. *Core Psychiatry*, 2nd edn. London: Saunders, 2005.

General revision

David A, Fleminger S, Kopelman M, Lovestone S, Mellers J. *Lishman's Organic Psychiatry: A Textbook of Neuropsychiatry*, 4th edn. Chichester: Wiley-Blackwell, 2009.

Fish FJ, Casey PR, Kelly B. *Fish's Clinical Psychopathology: Signs and Symptoms in Psychiatry*, 3rd edn. London: Royal College of Psychiatrists Publications, 2007.

Gross R. *Psychology: The Science of Mind and Behaviour*, 5th edn. London: Hodder Education, 2005.

Kumar P, Clark M. *Kumar and Clark's Clinical Medicine*, 7th edn. London: Saunders, 2009.

Stahl SM. *Stahl's Essential Psychopharmacology: Neuroscientific Basis and Practical Applications*, 3rd edn. Cambridge: Cambridge University Press, 2008.

Visual perception and sensory processes

1) Which of the following is true of figure–ground organization?
    a. Ground appears more solid than figure
    b. It is possible to see both organizations at the same time
    c. It is not reversible
    d. The larger an area or shape the more likely it is to be seen as figure
    e. Figure–ground relations can be perceived by senses other than vision

2) In the visual cortex:
    a. If a lesion occurs at the front, the fovea will suffer a scotoma
    b. The visual field map is upside down
    c. The left half of the visual field is mapped on to the left side
    d. The same region carries out both localization and recognition
    e. Each neuron is responsible for analysing a very large region of the image

3) Gestalt grouping determinants do not include:
    a. Ambiguity
    b. Proximity
    c. Similarity
    d. Continuation
    e. Closure

4) Which of the following is true of Gestalt grouping determinants?
    a. They create unstable forms within a given pattern
    b. They are not associated with reliable illusions
    c. They have no influence on perception
    d. They appear in audition
    e. Targets become more difficult to find as the similarity of non-targets increases

5) Monocular depth cues do not include:
    a. Relative height
    b. Proximity
    c. Interposition
    d. Linear perspective
    e. Motion parallax

6) Bottom-up processes:

    a. Are driven by a person's knowledge and expectations
    b. Underlie the powerful effects of contexts on our perception
    c. Help us perceive an ambiguous stimulus in more than one way
    d. Help us recognize the shape of an object on the basis of its geon description
    e. Play a major role in reading

7) Perceptual constancy:

    a. Enables us to determine how far away objects are
    b. Is a result of constancy in retinal images
    c. Makes localization difficult
    d. Cannot be eliminated by removing the object from its background
    e. Will not occur in senses other than vision

8) The eye movements used in scanning a picture:

    a. Are smooth and continuous
    b. Ensure that different parts of the picture will fall on to the fovea
    c. Use random fixation points
    d. Avoid selective attention
    e. All of the above

9) Which of the following is true of depth perception in infants?

    a. It begins to appear at about 1 month
    b. It is fully established by 6 months
    c. At 2 months, nearness is signalled by binocular disparity
    d. It is achieved with the establishment of monocular depth cues at 4 months
    e. It will be developed enough for reaching for the nearer of two objects at around 2 months

10) Perceptual constancy can be experienced for:

    a. Colour
    b. Shape
    c. Location
    d. Size
    e. All of the above

11) Cones:

    a. Are more sensitive to light than rods
    b. Respond to low levels of illumination
    c. Are more numerous
    d. Are for bright vision
    e. Are positioned more towards the periphery of the retina

12) With regard to colour perception, all of the following are true, except:

a. People with normal vision are dichromatic
b. Most colour deficiencies are genetic in origin
c. Colour blindness occurs more frequently in males
d. The colour blindness gene is recessive
e. The colour blindness gene is located in the X chromosome

13) Regarding perceptual set, all of the following are true, except:

a. Certain aspects of stimuli are perceived according to expectation
b. It is associated with a change in perception threshold
c. Perception is influenced by individual values
d. Perception is influenced by past experiences
e. Introverts cannot sustain attention for a long time

14) Gestalt psychology principles include all of the following, except:

a. The whole perception is the same as the sum of its parts
b. The percept corresponds to the simplest form in the pattern
c. The law of closure holds that partial outlines are perceived as whole
d. Adjacent items are grouped together
e. Figures are differentiated from ground by contours and boundaries, simulating objects

15) With regard to object constancy, all of the following are true, except:

a. Size constancy is present in a 4-month-old infant
b. Moving an object from close to the face to one metre away results in no apparent change in the size of the object, but retinal image size is reduced by half
c. To perceive an object moving, it is necessary for the image to move across the retina
d. Whatever the availability of light the colour of an object can be perceived
e. Emmett proposed the size–distance invariance principle

16) With regard to perceptual stimuli for various senses:

a. Absolute threshold is the minimum difference in stimulus magnitude necessary to tell two stimuli apart
b. A just noticeable difference is the minimum magnitude of a stimulus that can be reliably discriminated from no stimulus at all
c. The larger the value of the standard stimulus, the less sensitive the sensory system is to changes in intensity
d. Weber's law states that sensory perception is a logarithmic function of stimulus intensity
e. Fechner's law states that the increase in stimulus intensity needed to allow two sources of intensity to be perceived as being different is directly proportional to the value of the baseline intensity

Information processing and attention

17) Regarding information processing:
   a. Conceptually driven processing uses template matching
   b. Data-driven processing is applied when data are incomplete
   c. Data-driven processing uses perceptual schema
   d. Conceptually driven data can lead to misperceptions
   e. Data-driven processing biases the processing mechanisms to give expected results

18) Regarding attention, all of the following are true, except:
   a. The right frontal lobe is essential for the maintenance of attention
   b. In dichotic listening, the listener can switch rapidly to the unattended channel.
   c. In divided attention, loss of performance is called dual-task interference
   d. A defect in controlled attention might underlie symptoms of schizophrenia
   e. For controlled attention, little conscious effort is required

19) Illusions:
   a. Are less transient than hallucinations
   b. Do not need real stimuli
   c. Are not influenced by the perceptual set
   d. Suggest an active search for meaning
   e. Have no emotional component

20) Disturbance of depth perception and perceptual constancy is seen in all of the following, except:
   a. Schizophrenia
   b. Depersonalization
   c. Obsessive compulsive disorder
   d. Delirium
   e. Epilepsy

21) Signal detection theory states that perception depends on all of the following, except:
   a. Stimulus intensity
   b. Stroop effect
   c. Motivation
   d. Previous experience
   e. Expectations

Motivation, emotion and stress

22) Regarding integration of hunger signals in the hypothalamus, all of the following are true, except:

   a. A lesion in the lateral hypothalamus produces lack of hunger
   b. A lesion in the ventromedial hypothalamus produces a voracious appetite
   c. Morphine can suppress appetite when it is injected into the ventro-medial hypothalamus
   d. Amphetamine can suppress appetite when it is injected into the lateral hypothalamus
   e. Lesions in the mesolimbic dopamine system mimic a lesion in the lateral hypothalamus

23) With regard to intrinsic motivation theories, all of the following are true, except:

   a. Attachment is a result of intrinsic primary drive
   b. High arousal leads to increased performance
   c. Cognitive dissonance theory was first formulated by Festinger
   d. Need for achievement theory was formulated by McClelland
   e. If two or more inconsistent cognitions are held simultaneously, discomfort occurs

24) With regard to intrinsic motivation theories, all of the following are true, except:

   a. The activity engaged in has its own intrinsic reward
   b. A moderate degree of arousal leads to an optimum degree of alertness
   c. The Yerkes–Dodson curve is U-shaped
   d. The individual motivated to achieve cognitive consistency may change one or more of the cognitions
   e. When attitude and behaviour are inconsistent, the alteration of attitude brings cognitive consistency

25) Maslow's hierarchy of needs includes all of the following, except:

   a. Self-actualization
   b. Self-motivation
   c. Self-esteem
   d. Safety
   e. Physical needs

26) Regarding motivation, all of the following are true, except:

   a. Reward is mediated by the mesolimbic dopaminergic system
   b. Maslow's hierarchy of needs states that needs at one level should be satisfied before the next level becomes important
   c. Gender differences are observed in need for achievement
   d. Motivation is mainly a result of primary reinforcers
   e. Need for achievement theory explains pleasure resulting from mastery

27) Cognitive dissonance:

   a. Is affectively neutral
   b. Helps us find choices in uncertain situations
   c. Decreases with personal responsibility for actions
   d. Cannot be reduced by denying information
   e. Is the same as attitude-discrepant behaviour

28) Regarding theories of emotion, all of the following are true, except:

   a. The James–Lange theory views the emotional response to a situation as resulting from physiological factors
   b. The Cannon–Bard theory holds that following perception of an emotionally important event, both somatic experience and the experience of emotion occur together
   c. Schacter's cognitive labelling theory states that emotional experience is based on cognitive appraisal of the arousal
   d. On a Yerkes–Dodson curve the optimal level is a fixed point regardless of task complexity
   e. According to the Schachter and Singer model, cognitive cues are important in interpretation of arousal

29) Regarding stress:

   a. Stimulus models take into account the person interacting with the environment
   b. Response models view stress as the non-specific response of the body to the demands placed upon it
   c. Response models take into account the psychological reactions to stress
   d. The general adaptation syndrome includes alarm reaction, resistance and relaxation
   e. In transactional models the individual is not seen as an active participant in the process of emotional appraisal

30) Physiological reactions to stress include all of the following, except:

   a. Increased metabolic rate
   b. Increased heart rate
   c. Constriction of pupil
   d. Secretion of endorphins and ACTH
   e. Release of extra sugar from the liver

31) Regarding stress, all of the following are true, except:
   a. Positive events can be stressful
   b. Assault victims are twice as likely to develop mental health problems at some time after the assault
   c. The more uncontrollable the event seems, the less likely it is to be perceived as stressful
   d. Predictability of the occurrence of a stressful event reduces the severity of the stress
   e. Employed mothers are more likely to develop heart disease

32) Regarding stress, all of the following are true, except:
   a. Type A personality was described by Friedman and Rosenman
   b. Type A personality is related to increased proneness to heart attack
   c. It is possible to modify type A personality
   d. Type B personality strives for achievement with time urgency
   e. Several studies have found that a person's level of hostility is a better predictor of heart attack than the person's overall level of type A behaviour

33) Regarding locus of control, all of the following are true, except:
   a. It was proposed by Rotter
   b. The more anxious or depressed a person, the more internal his or her locus of control tends to be
   c. A greater external locus of control is associated with a greater vulnerability to physical illness
   d. With successful therapeutic intervention locus of control can be changed
   e. Biofeedback aims to change the physiological state directly

34) The following defence mechanisms used to cope with stress are all correctly matched, except:
   a. Denial−Concentration only on the current task
   b. Projection−Empathy
   c. Rationalization−Substitution of other thoughts for disturbing ones
   d. Repression−Suppression of inappropriate feelings
   e. Isolation−Objectivity

35) Regarding learned helplessness:
   a. It was proposed by Rotter
   b. Those who believe nobody could have controlled the outcome of the event are more likely to develop learned helplessness
   c. Locus of control theory is largely based on this concept
   d. It develops regardless of a person's attribution
   e. It may explain why some women remain in abusive relationships even when they have opportunities to leave

Memory, language and thought

36) In memory:

   a. The regions in the right hemisphere of the brain are activated during encoding
   b. The regions in the left hemisphere of the brain are activated during retrieval
   c. Immediate memory and working memory are synonymous
   d. Short-term memory has a duration of 20 seconds unless it is rehearsed
   e. Sensory or iconic memory plays a major role in thought and conscious recollection

37) With regard to brain regions involved in memory:

   a. The hippocampus is critical for long-term memory and working memory
   b. The frontal cortex is critical for long-term memory
   c. People with medial temporal lobe damage have severe amnesia and have difficulty remembering material for more than a few seconds
   d. People with medial temporal lobe damage have severe amnesia and have difficulty recognizing familiar people
   e. People with medial temporal lobe damage have an abnormal working memory

38) In human memory, all of the following are true, except:

   a. Encoding is mainly acoustic
   b. Visual encoding rapidly fades
   c. Sensory memory is long lived
   d. Haptic memory is a sensory memory
   e. Sensory memory is retained in an unprocessed form in peripheral receptors

39) In working memory, all of the following are true, except:

   a. Rehearsal facilitates phonological coding
   b. Eidetic memory occurs mainly in children
   c. Acoustic and visual–spatial buffers are mediated by the same brain structures
   d. The capacity of working memory is 7 ± 2
   e. Chunking improves the capacity of working memory

40) Regarding working memory, all of the following are true, except:

   a. It can be boosted by regrouping
   b. It can be boosted by displacement
   c. It can be boosted by chunking
   d. It can be boosted by rehearsing
   e. Forgetting may occur due to decay

41) About memory, all of the following are true, except:

   a. The recency effect is remembering easily the most recent words encountered from a list of words
   b. The primacy effect is retrieving the first words on a word list
   c. Both primacy and recency effects are involved in remembering a list of words
   d. The serial position effect is retrieving the last few words on a word list
   e. The recency effect is explained by the short time elapsed before recall

42) Regarding short-term memory:

   a. Encoding is mainly acoustic
   b. Verbal short-term memory is stored in the left hemisphere and visual short-term memory is stored in the right hemisphere
   c. Retrieval is effortless and error free
   d. Short-term memory has an average limit of seven pieces of information
   e. All of the above are true

43) Which of the following is true of semantic memory?

   a. It is a long-term memory for events
   b. It is autobiographical in nature
   c. It is stored in terms of meaning
   d. Semantic encoding is less efficient than rehearsal
   e. It is continually changing

44) Which of the following is true of forgetting?

   a. It is mainly caused by storage failure
   b. Retrieval failure can explain the 'tip-of-the-tongue' experience
   c. Forgetting by interference is not item dependent
   d. Forgetting by decay is item dependent
   e. All of the above

45) With regard to language units and processes, all of the following are true, except:

   a. All languages have the same set of phonemes
   b. Morpheme refers to any small linguistic unit that carries meaning
   c. Words, prefixes and suffixes are examples of morphemes
   d. Over the first year of life children learn which phonemes are relevant to their language and lose their ability to discriminate between other phonemes.
   e. The first step in extracting propositions from a complex sentence is to deconstruct the sentence into phrases

46) Regarding the development of language:

   a. Children learn language by imitating adults
   b. Children acquire language through conditioning
   c. Children form a hypothesis about a rule of language, test it and retain it if it works
   d. There is indirect evidence for the existence of a critical period for language acquisition, in the case of children who have experienced extreme isolation
   e. All of the above

47) As a building block of thought, concept:

   a. Represents an entire class
   b. Is an example of the brain's ability to reduce information-processing load
   c. Allows prediction
   d. May include physical objects
   e. All of the above

48) Prototypes:

   a. Are the most logical and strictly accurate examples of a member of a concept
   b. Represent the most popular and best recognized example
   c. Cannot be accessed easily
   d. Are a more perfect indicator of the concept than its core properties
   e. Are not universal

49) About acquiring concepts, all of the following are true, except:

   a. Explicit teaching is likely to be the means by which we learn cores of concepts
   b. Experience seems to be the usual means by which we acquire prototypes
   c. Five-year-old children show a clear shift from the prototype to the core as the final arbitrator of concept decisions
   d. Prior knowledge may affect every aspect of concept attainment
   e. Research shows that prototype-based categorization does not depend on the brain structures that mediate long-term memory

50) In reasoning, all of the following are true, except:

   a. In deductively valid arguments, it is impossible for the conclusion of the argument to be false if its premises are true
   b. Inductive reasoning is probabilistic
   c. An algorithm, if applied stepwise, will always guarantee the solution to a problem
   d. Heuristics invariably yield the correct answer
   e. Heuristic arguments depend on cognitive short-cuts such as prototypes

1) e.

Figure appears more solid; the smaller area is seen as figure.

2) b.

A lesion at the back causes foveal scotoma; the map of the visual field is upside down and mirror reversed; localization is in the posterior parietal and recognition in the inferior temporal.

3) a.

The determinants (b−e) proposed by Gestalt psychologists create the most stable, consistent and simple forms.

4) d.

Stable forms are associated with reliable illusions; targets are easier to find as the similarity of non-targets increases.

5) b.

Monocular cues also include shading and shadows.

6) d.

a, b, c and e are top-down processes.

7) a.

Impressions on the retina change; perceptual constancy makes localization easy, can be eliminated, and may occur in other senses, e.g. hearing.

8) b.

Eye movements when scanning a picture consist of successive fixations on points that convey most information about the picture.

9) b.

Depth perception begins to appear at 2−3 months; at 4 months, nearness is signalled by binocular disparity; monocular depth cues are established at 6 months; reaching for the nearer of two objects begins at 4 months.

10) e.

Perceptual constancy is the tendency for the appearance of objects to remain constant even though their impression on the retina is changing.

11) d.

a, b, c and e apply to rods.

12) a.
People with normal vision are described as trichomates and they can match a wide range of colours with three primary colours. Dichromates are individuals with deficient colour vision who can match only two primary colours. Monochromates are individuals with deficient colour vision who are unable to discriminate between the different wavelengths of colours.

13) e.
Introverts can sustain attention for a long time.

14) a.
The whole perception is different from the sum of its parts.

15) c.
In stroboscopic motion and induced motion, the image does not move on the retina.

16) c.
(a) Just noticeable difference, (b) absolute threshold, (d) Fechner's, (e) Weber's.

17) d.
Data-driven processing uses template matching. Conceptually driven processing is applied when data are incomplete; it uses perceptual schema and biases the processing.

18) e.
For automatic attention little conscious effort is required, but for controlled attention more effort is needed.

19) d.
Illusions are more transient, need real stimuli, are influenced by the perceptual set, and have a strong emotional component.

20) c.
In temporal lobe epilepsy and acute brain syndromes disturbance of perception occurs.

Puri B, Hall A. Chapter 4. In: *Revision Notes in Psychiatry*, 2nd edn. London: Arnold/Hodder Education, 2004.

21) b.
Automatic processing interferes with controlled processing.

22) c.
Morphine can stimulate feeding when it is injected into the ventromedial hypothalamus.

23) b.
High and low arousals lead to reduced performance, and moderate arousal is optimum (Yerkes–Dodson curve).

24) c.
The Yerkes–Dodson curve is an inverted U-shape.

25) b.
Love and belonging, and autonomy are also included.

26) d.
Motivation is mainly a result of secondary reinforcers.

27) b.
Cognitive dissonance can cause discomfort and dysphoria, increases with personal responsibility, and can be reduced by denying information.

28) d.
On the Yerkes–Dodson curve the optimal level is not a fixed point and depends on many factors, including task complexity.

29) b.
Stimulus models take no account of the person interacting with the environment. Response models do not take into account the psychological reactions to stress. The general adaptation syndrome includes alarm reaction, resistance and exhaustion.

30) c.
Pupil dilation is the physiological reaction associated with stress. Increased blood pressure also occurs in association with stress.

31) c.
The more uncontrollable the event seems the more likely it is to be perceived as stressful. Employed women are not at high risk of CHD but employed mothers are at higher risk.

32) d.
Type A personality: competitiveness, difficulty relaxing, impatience, anger, striving for achievement with time urgency.

33) b.
The more anxious or depressed a person, the more external his or her locus of control tends to be.

34) c.
Rationalization–Logical analysis; Reaction formation–Substitution of other thoughts for disturbing ones.

35) e.
Learned helplessness was proposed by Seligman. Those who believe nobody could have controlled the outcome of the event are less likely to develop learned helplessness, while those who believe they have personal control over the event are more likely to develop learned helplessness; the cognitive theory of depression is largely based on this concept.

Seligman MEP. *Helplessness: On Depression, Development, and Death.* San Francisco: WH Freeman, 1975.

36) d.
The right hemisphere of the brain is used for retrieval; the left hemisphere is used for encoding; iconic memory plays far less of a role in thought and conscious recollection.

37) d.
The hippocampus is critical for long-term memory only and not for working memory. The frontal cortex is critical in working memory. Medial temporal lobe damage does not affect working memory.

38) c.
Sensory memory is short lived.

39) c.
Acoustic buffer is mediated by the left hemisphere; visual–spatial buffers are mediated by the right hemisphere.

40) b.
Displacement is a cause of forgetting.

41) d.
Serial position effect means that items from the intermediate position are least likely to be recalled.

42) e.
Short-term memory is temporary working memory; it is lost in 20 seconds unless it is rehearsed; it uses the principles of displacement, chunking, primacy effect, recency effect and eidetic memory.

43) c.
a, b and e apply to episodic memory.

44) b.
Forgetting is mainly due to retrieval failure; forgetting by interference is item dependent and by decay is time dependent.

45) a.
Every language has a different set of phonemes. A phoneme is a speech sound. The English language has 40 phonemes.

46) e.
Research has shown that there is a critical period for learning syntax.

47) e.
Categorization refers to the process of assigning an object to a concept.

48) b.
Prototypes are not necessarily logical or even strictly accurate examples of a member of a concept, but represent the most popular and best recognized example. They can be accessed easily, and are highly salient examples of a concept, but these properties are not necessarily conditions for concept membership, whereas the core properties are more central to concept membership. For some concepts culture has a major impact on the prototype, but for more natural concepts prototypes are surprisingly universal.

49) c.
Not until age 10 do children show a clear shift from the prototype to the core as the final arbitrator of concept decisions.

Keil FC, Batterman N. A characteristic-to-defining shift in the acquisition of word meaning. *J Verb Learn Verb Behav* 1984; **23**: 221–36.

50) d.
A heuristic procedure is a short-cut that is relatively easy to apply and can often yield the correct answer, but not invariably so.

Further reading

Munafo M. *Psychology for the MRCPsych*, 2nd edn. London: Hodder Education, 2002.
Puri B, Hall A. Chapters 1–4. In: *Revision Notes in Psychiatry*, 2nd edn. London: Arnold/Hodder Education, 2004.
Smith EE, Bem DJ, Nolen-Hoeksema S. Chapters 2–6. In: *Atkinson and Hilgard's Introduction to Psychology*, 14th edn. Florence, KY: Wadsworth Publishing Company, 2003.

2. Learning theory and personality: Questions

Learning theory

1) Learning:
   a. Is a temporary change in observable behaviour
   b. Does not require prior experience
   c. Includes behavioural changes caused by maturation
   d. Includes behavioural changes due to drug effects
   e. Does not include behavioural changes due to hunger

2) In Pavlov's experiments:
   a. Salivation was an unconditioned stimulus before conditioning
   b. Salivation was a conditioned stimulus after conditioning
   c. Food was a conditioned stimulus after conditioning
   d. Light was a conditioned stimulus after conditioning
   e. None of the above is correct

3) Regarding classical conditioning, all of the following are true, except:
   a. The conditioned response is an acquired response to a conditioned stimulus
   b. The acquisition stage is the period in which an association is acquired between conditioned stimulus and conditioned response
   c. In delayed conditioning the onset of the conditioned stimulus precedes that of an unconditioned stimulus
   d. In delayed conditioning the conditioned stimulus continues until the response occurs
   e. Delayed conditioning is optimal when the delay between the onset of the two stimuli is around half a second

4) In classical conditioning:
   a. The subject is active in learning
   b. Response is typically autonomic or emotional
   c. Spontaneous recovery is stronger than a conditioned response
   d. The longer the time between extinction and reappearance, the weaker is the response
   e. The strength of the conditioned response is inversely proportional to the intensity of the stimulus

5) Regarding classical conditioning, all of the following are true, except:

    a. Forward conditioning: conditioned stimulus (CS) comes first, and while it is still happening the unconditioned stimulus (UCS) occurs
    b. Simultaneous conditioning: CS and UCS occur at the same time
    c. Trace conditioning: CS comes first, and after it stops UCS occurs
    d. Backward conditioning: CS occurs after UCS has started
    e. Delayed conditioning: CS occurs after UCS has started and stops before UCS stops

6) Which of the following is true of extinction?

    a. It occurs in both classical and operant conditioning
    b. It is the same as forgetting
    c. Usually the complete loss of the conditioned stimulus occurs
    d. Merely not presenting the conditioned stimulus will result in the extinction of the conditioned response after some time.
    e. Relearning of extinguished associations is usually slower than learning in controls

7) Regarding generalization:

    a. It accounts in part for an individual's ability to react to novel stimuli that are similar to familiar ones
    b. It occurs frequently in everyday life
    c. The response will vary in strength as a function of similarity
    d. It is a stimulus similar to the original stimulus eliciting the conditioned response
    e. All of the above

8) Which of the following is true of discrimination in classical conditioning?

    a. It is a reaction to differences
    b. When distinguishing similar but different stimuli one is reinforced and the other is not
    c. It is brought about through differential association
    d. It can be achieved through differential reinforcement
    e. All of the above

9) With regard to incubation, all of the following are true, except:

    a. The increase in strength of conditioned response results from repeated brief exposure to the conditioned stimulus
    b. It could explain how phobias are perpetuated
    c. A reduction in the emotional response as a result of escape from a phobic object is a negative reinforcement leading to incubation
    d. It was demonstrated by Watson and Rayner in the Little Albert experiment
    e. The incubation theory of phobic fear was proposed by Eysenck

10) In learning theory:

   a. Stimulus preparedness means that specific objects like blood and snakes are much more likely to be the subject of phobias than others
   b. Temporal contiguity between the conditioned stimulus and unconditioned stimulus is the most important factor in the development of classical conditioning
   c. In classical conditioning, conditioned responses are likely to be of greater magnitude than unconditioned responses
   d. A higher-order conditioning uses a conditioned response as an unconditioned stimulus
   e. The learning occurs only if the subject's behaviour is reinforced

11) Regarding operant conditioning, all of the following are true, except:

   a. Thorndike described operant and respondent behaviours
   b. A voluntary behaviour is engaged in because its occurrence is reinforced by being rewarded
   c. A voluntary behaviour independent of stimuli is termed operant behaviour
   d. A behaviour that is dependent on known stimuli is termed respondent behaviour
   e. Thorndike's law of effect holds that voluntary behaviour that is paired with subsequent reward is strengthened

12) Regarding positive reinforcement, all of the following are true, except:

   a. It is synonymous with reward
   b. It is a pleasant stimulus that follows a desired behaviour
   c. It increases the likelihood of the desired behaviour
   d. Allowing a child to leave his room only when he is no longer having a temper tantrum is an example
   e. A high grade on an examination is an example

13) Removal of an unpleasant stimulus after a desired behaviour occurs is:

   a. Positive reinforcement
   b. Negative reinforcement
   c. Positive punishment
   d. Negative punishment
   e. Primary reinforcement

14) Regarding types of reinforcement and punishment, all of the following are true, except:
   a. Negative reinforcement increases the likelihood of the desired behaviour
   b. Negative punishment is removal of a pleasant stimulus after a desired behaviour occurs
   c. Positive punishment is presentation of an unpleasant stimulus after an undesired behaviour occurs
   d. Positive punishment decreases the likelihood of the undesired behaviour
   e. Negative punishment decreases the likelihood of the undesired behaviour

15) Regarding reinforcement, all of the following are true, except:
   a. Primary reinforcers are those stimuli that meet biological needs
   b. Secondary reinforcers are those that one has to learn the value of
   c. Punishment tends not to be so effective in learning situations as positive or negative reinforcers
   d. In continuous reinforcement, reinforcement takes place following every conditioned response
   e. Continuous reinforcement is not good at maintaining a high response rate

16) With regard to conditioning, all of the following are true, except:
   a. In avoidance conditioning, fear reduction is a positive reinforcement
   b. Avoidance conditioning demonstrates principles of both classical and operant conditioning
   c. Escape conditioning is a variety of negative conditioning
   d. When it is learnt, escape from an aversive stimulus is very resistant to extinction
   e. An extreme punishment may elicit aggressive behaviour that is more serious than the original undesirable behaviour

17) In partial reinforcement, all of the following are true, except:
   a. Fixed interval schedule is poor in maintaining the conditioned response
   b. Variable interval schedule is very good in maintaining the conditioned response
   c. Fixed ratio schedule is very poor in maintaining a high response rate
   d. Variable ratio schedule is very good in maintaining a high response rate
   e. Variable ratio schedule is more likely to produce emotional outbursts during the learning phase

18) Behavioural explanation of the aetiology of phobias includes all of the following, except:

    a. Habituation
    b. Stimulus preparedness
    c. Incubation
    d. Escape conditioning
    e. Avoidance conditioning

19) Reciprocal inhibition:

    a. Is based on Wolpe's principle
    b. Is used to treat conditions associated with anticipatory anxiety
    c. Is based on the concept that desired and undesired behaviours are incompatible, which facilitates changes in the desired direction
    d. Is used in systematic desensitization
    e. All of the above

20) Habituation is:

    a. An example of counter-conditioning
    b. Applied in systematic desensitization
    c. Applied in exposure and response prevention
    d. The process by which an organism learns to weaken its reaction to a weak stimulus that has no serious consequences
    e. All of the above

21) All of the following are paired correctly, except:

    a. Flooding—Enforced exposure
    b. Modelling—Vicarious exposure
    c. Chaining—Complex behaviour learned in separate steps
    d. Shaping—Explains behavioural disturbances in learning disability
    e. Cueing—Based on operant conditioning

22) All of the following are components of Bandura's observational learning model, except:

    a. Attention
    b. Perception
    c. Generalization
    d. Memory
    e. Motivation

23) In observational learning:

    a. Symbolic modelling is more effective than live modelling
    b. The concept of reciprocal determinism is important
    c. Modelling cannot be used in a group setting
    d. Principles of classical and operant conditioning are excluded
    e. All of the above

24) With regard to cognitive learning, which of the following statements are true?

a. The cognitive map is associated with Tolman's model
b. The concept of insight learning is associated with Kohler
c. Complex learning occurs in two phases
d. Complex learning is intimately related to memory and thinking
e. All of the above

25) In psychoanalytic models of learning, all of the following are true, except:

a. Behaviour is determined by intrapsychic processes
b. Problem behaviour is the focus of the study and the treatment
c. Childhood experiences are the focus of analysis
d. Problem behaviour is a symptom of unconscious conflict
e. Subjective methods of interpretation of behaviour are used

26) In the behavioural model of learning, all of the following are true, except:

a. Behaviour is determined by current contingencies
b. Behaviour is determined by reinforcement history
c. Behaviour is determined by genetic endowment
d. Behaviour is determined by intrapsychic processes
e. Behaviour is determined by needs deriving from basic drives

27) Functional analysis in behavioural therapy includes all of the following, except:

a. A direct record of the frequency of occurrence of the behaviour studied
b. A direct record of the duration of occurrence of the behaviour studied
c. A direct record of the intensity of the behaviour studied
d. A direct record of the defence mechanisms in the behaviour studied
e. A direct record of the stimuli increasing the incidence of the behaviour studied

28) Optimal conditions for observational learning include:

a. The behaviour observed is being reinforced
b. Perceived similarity
c. Active participation
d. Familiarity of the model
e. All of the above

29) All of the following are true about modelling, except:

    a. It can improve self-efficacy
    b. It can decrease aggression
    c. It can eliminate negative behaviour patterns and decrease anxiety threshold
    d. It can be used in weight-reduction programmes
    e. It cannot lower the pain threshold

30) All of the following are true, except:

    a. Observational learning can occur without reinforcement
    b. When a person dislikes a model, imitative behaviour is less likely to occur
    c. Insight learning does not require understanding of the relationship between various elements of the problem to be solved
    d. Latent learning is manifested when there is a need to satisfy a basic drive
    e. According to tension reduction theory, people are completely unaware of their avoidance patterns

31) All of the following names are correctly paired with their associated theories, except:

    a. Wolpe—Anxiety hierarchy
    b. Dollard and Miller—Tension reduction theory
    c. Beck—Learned helplessness model of depression
    d. Kandel—Habituation and sensitization
    e. Harlow—Learning set

32) Regarding imprinting, all of the following are true, except:

    a. It is an ethological concept
    b. It was described by Lorenz
    c. It is an important component of behavioural treatment of phobias
    d. It is normally species specific
    e. All of the above

33) Regarding application of learning theory in behavioural psychology, all of the following are true, except:

    a. Only a quarter of animal phobias are associated with prior traumatic experience with animals
    b. We may be prepared to acquire certain fears on evolutionary grounds
    c. Exposure therapy for anxiety disorders depends on habituation
    d. Self-exposure should be attempted only with intense supervision from the therapist
    e. More effective exposure occurs in real life than in the imagination

34) With regard to behavioural therapy, all of the following are true, except:

    a. For specific phobias, 70–80% of patients are successfully treated
    b. For agoraphobia, exposure has been shown to be more effective than waiting and attention controls, and as effective as medication
    c. The combination of exposure and high-dose benzodiazepines is more effective for agoraphobia than exposure alone
    d. In the short term, antidepressants plus exposure are the most effective treatment for panic and agoraphobia
    e. Meta-analytic studies have shown exposure to be a more effective treatment for social phobia

35) Functional behaviour assessment includes:

    a. Exploration of the childhood origins of antecedents
    b. Family history and dynamics
    c. Expressed emotions in the family
    d. An understanding of incubation
    e. Assessment of the patient's projection

36) The following clinical applications of behaviour therapy are all correctly paired, except:

    a. Agoraphobia–Graded exposure and flooding
    b. Alcohol dependence–Exposure and response prevention
    c. Schizophrenia–The token economy procedure
    d. Post-traumatic stress disorder (PTSD)–Eye movement desensitization and reprocessing (EMDR)
    e. Type A behaviour–Biofeedback

37) With regard to aversion therapy, all of the following are true, except:

    a. A noxious stimulus is presented immediately after a specific behavioural response
    b. Covert sensitization is a form of behaviour therapy in which an undesirable behaviour is paired with an unpleasant image in order to eliminate that behaviour
    c. Aversion therapy can be used to treat behaviours with impulsive qualities
    d. Punishment always leads to the expected decrease in response
    e. Punishment can sometimes be positively reinforcing

38) With regard to application of learning principles to treatment, all of the following are true, except:

   a. In systematic desensitization, the learned relaxation state and the anxiety-provoking scenes are systematically paired in the treatment
   b. In systematic desensitization, a conditioned stimulus is used to avoid an unconditioned painful stimulus
   c. Stimulus preparedness of some phobias may make them more difficult to treat
   d. Response prevention is characteristically combined with flooding
   e. Implosion is flooding achieved in the imagination rather than in real life

39) In learning and conditioning:

   a. Operant conditioning is contingent on a particular stimulus
   b. Punishment contingent upon response leads to learned helplessness
   c. In operant conditioning, the behaviour preceding the reinforcer always alters in frequency
   d. Counter-conditioning and reciprocal inhibition are involved in systematic desensitization
   e. Habituation explains generalization

40) All of the following are related to aetiology and maintenance of phobias, except:

   a. Avoidance learning
   b. Seligman's preparedness theory
   c. Stimulus generalization
   d. Magnification and minimization
   e. Fear of castration

41) All of the following are involved in the aetiology and maintenance of agoraphobia, except:

   a. Avoidance conditioning
   b. Escape conditioning
   c. Sensitization
   d. Over-inclusion
   e. Incubation

42) With regard to application of learning principles:

   a. Vicarious learning involves extinction
   b. In a behavioural assessment it is important to understand the patient's projections
   c. Classical conditioning explains how anxiety arises in response to environmental stimuli
   d. Learned helplessness is an example of classical conditioning
   e. In operant conditioning, the reinforcer precedes the behaviour

Personality

43) Regarding Eysenck's contribution to personality theories, all of the following are true, except:

   a. The personality dimensions extroversion, neuroticism and psychoticism are normally distributed
   b. Extroversion exists as a balance between excitation and inhibition processes in the ascending reticular activating system
   c. Neuroticism is connected to the reactivity of the autonomic nervous system
   d. Eysenck's Personality Inventory is a self-reported questionnaire to assess the three personality dimensions
   e. Eysenck's Personality Inventory contains an index assessing response bias

44) Regarding personality theories, all of the following are correct, except:

   a. Cattell used factor analytic studies
   b. Allport described common traits and individual traits
   c. Kelly's personal construct theory proposes that the construct system is hierarchically organized
   d. Bannister devised the Construct Repertory Test
   e. Q-sort technique is devised from a theory based on Rogers's client-centred therapy

45) Regarding the psychoanalytic approach to personality structure, all of the following are true, except:

   a. In Freud's structural model of the mind, all of the id is submerged in the unconscious
   b. In Freud's structural model of the mind, most of the ego is submerged in the unconscious
   c. In Freud's structural model of the mind, most of the superego is in the conscious or in the preconscious
   d. A child resolves the oedipal conflict by identifying with the same-sex parent
   e. Recent psychodynamic theorists believe that ego performs other functions besides finding ways to satisfy id impulses, including learning how to cope with the environment and making sense of experience

46) Carl Rogers:

    a. Introduced non-directive psychotherapy
    b. Believed that individuals have an innate tendency to move toward growth, maturity and positive change, described as actualizing tendency
    c. Argued that people are likely to function more effectively if they feel they are valued by their parents regardless of their feelings, attitudes and behaviours
    d. Described the form of psychotherapy in which the therapist's role is to act as a sounding board while the client explores and analyses his or her own problems
    e. All of the above

47) Regarding cognitive approaches of personality theories, all of the following are true, except:

    a. According to Kelly, personal constructs take an either/or form
    b. Differences in self-schemas produce differences in behaviour
    c. A person whose self-schema includes being physically fit is less likely to exercise regularly
    d. According to Bem's gender-schema theory, individuals who describe themselves as having both masculine and feminine traits are referred to as androgynous
    e. None of the above

Levels of awareness

48) All of the following are true about sleep stages, except:

    a. Most REM sleep occurs in the last part of the night
    b. Sleepers who are awakened during REM sleep report a dream about 50% of the time
    c. During NREM sleep, heart and breathing rates decrease markedly
    d. During REM sleep, the body is almost paralysed, except the muscles of the vital organs
    e. In REM sleep, the metabolic rate of the brain increases somewhat compared with during wakefulness

49) All of the following statements are true about the pattern of variation of sleep cycle with age, except:

    a. Newborn infants spend half their sleeping time in REM sleep
    b. The proportion of REM sleep drops to 20–25% of total sleep time by age 5 and remains fairly constant until old age
    c. Older people tend to experience more stage 3 and 4 sleep
    d. REM sleep drops to 18% or less at old age
    e. A natural kind of insomnia sets in as people grow older

50) In the sleep–wake cycle:
    a. In REM sleep, the brain is largely isolated from its sensory and motor channels
    b. The dreams reported when a person is roused from REM sleep tend to be visually vivid, with emotional and illogical features.
    c. The longer the period of REM sleep before arousal, the longer and more elaborate is the reported dream.
    d. NREM dreams are more directly related to what is happening in the person's waking life.
    e. All of the above are true

51) Regarding states of consciousness, all of the following are true, except:
    a. Narcolepsy is regarded as the intrusion of REM episodes into daytime hours
    b. Some people are more readily hypnotized than others, although most people show some susceptibility
    c. Reduction of pain is one of the beneficial uses of hypnosis
    d. Sleep spindles and K complexes occur in stage 4 sleep
    e. Penile erection is common in REM sleep

2. Learning theory and personality: Answers

1) e.
Learning is a relatively permanent change, from prior experience, and does not include changes through maturation and temporary conditions like drug effects, hunger, fatigue, etc.

2) d.
Salivation was an unconditioned response before the conditioning, and a conditioned response after conditioning. Food was an unconditioned stimulus.

3) b.
The acquisition stage is the period in which an association is acquired between conditioned stimulus and unconditioned stimulus.

4) b.
The subject is passive; spontaneous recovery is weaker than conditioned response; the longer the time between extinction and reappearance, the stronger is the response; the strength of the conditioned response is directly proportional to the intensity of the stimulus.

5) e.
Delayed conditioning is the same as forward conditioning.

6) a.
Extinction is not the same as forgetting; partial recovery occurs; it needs repeat presentation of a conditioned stimulus without an unconditioned stimulus; relearning is quicker.

7) e.
Generalization is a process whereby once a conditioned response has been established to a given stimulus, that response is evoked by a similar stimulus. The strength of response is inversely proportional to the difference between two stimuli.

8) e.
Discrimination is the differential recognition of and response to two or more similar stimuli.

9) d.
Watson and Rayner demonstrated generalization in the Little Albert experiment.

10) a.

A higher predictability, that is a higher probability of unconditioned stimulus occurring with conditioned stimulus, is more important than temporal contiguity. Conditioned responses are lesser in magnitude. A higher-order conditioning uses a conditioned stimulus as an unconditioned stimulus. Vicarious learning occurs without reinforcement.

11) a.

Skinner described operant and respondent behaviours.

12) d.

Allowing a child to leave his room when he is no longer having a temper tantrum is an example of negative reinforcement.

13) b.

A negative reinforcer is an aversive stimulus whose removal increases the probability of occurrence of the operant behaviour. Punishment is the situation that occurs if an aversive stimulus is presented whenever the given behaviour occurs, thereby reducing the probability of occurrence of this response.

14) b.

Negative punishment is the removal of a pleasant stimulus after an undesired behaviour occurs.

15) e.

Continuous reinforcement leads to the maximum response rate.

16) a.

In avoidance conditioning, fear reduction is a negative reinforcement.

17) c.

In partial reinforcement, only some of the conditioned responses are reinforced. Fixed ratio schedule is good in maintaining a high response rate.

18) a.

Habituation is an important principle of behavioural treatment of obsessive compulsive disorder.

19) e.

The theory of reciprocal inhibition is used to treat phobias through counter-conditioning.

20) e.

Habituation is used in treatment of obsessive compulsive disorder.

21) d.
Shaping is used to manage behavioural disturbances in learning disability.

22) c.
Generalization is a component of associative learning.

23) b.
Live modelling is more effective than symbolic modelling. Modelling is used in group settings in psychotherapy; it includes principles of both classical and operant conditioning.

24) e.
Complex learning occurs in two phases: insight learning and latent learning.

25) b.
In the behavioural model, problem behaviour is the focus of the study and the treatment, and in the psychoanalytic model the underlying unconscious conflict is the focus of the treatment.

26) d.
Intrapsychic processes are part of psychoanalytic models.

27) d.
Functional analysis in behavioural therapy does not include recording of defence mechanisms.

28) e.
Observational learning can occur without direct reinforcement.

29) e.
Modelling can lower the pain threshold.

30) c.
Insight learning is based on prior understanding.

31) c.
Beck is associated with the cognitive triad and Seligman with the learned helplessness model of depression.

32) c.
An example of imprinting is that a goose follows the first moving object it sees after it hatches.

33) d.
Only 23% of animal phobias are associated with prior traumatic experience with animals (McNally & Steketee 1985); many patients can carry out self-exposure effectively with intervention only from the therapist; more effective exposure occurs in real life than in the imagination (Emmelkamp & Wessels 1975).

Emmelkamp PM, Wessels H. Flooding in imagination vs. flooding in vivo: A comparison with agoraphobics. *Behav Res Ther* 1975; **13**: 7–15.
McNally RJ, Steketee GS. The etiology and maintenance of severe animal phobias. *Behav Res Ther* 1985; **23**: 431–5.

34) c.
Exposure has been shown to be more effective than waiting and attention controls (DeRubeis & Crits-Cristoph 1998); the combination of exposure and high-dose benzodiazepines is less effective for agoraphobia than exposure alone (Marks et al 1993); antidepressants plus exposure are the most effective treatment (van Balkom et al 1997); meta-analytic studies have shown exposure to be a more effective treatment for social phobia (Chambless and Gillis 1993).

Chambless DL, Gillis MM. Cognitive therapy of anxiety disorders. *J Consult Clin Psychol* 1993; **61**: 248–60.
DeRubeis RJ, Crits-Christoph P. Empirically supported individual and group psychological treatments for adult mental disorders. *J Consult Clin Psychol* 1998; **66**: 37–52.
Marks IM, Swinson RP, Basoglu M, et al. Alprazolam and exposure alone and combined in panic disorder with agoraphobia. A controlled study in London and Toronto. *Br J Psychiatry* 1993; **162**: 776–87.
van Balkom AJLM, Bakker A, Spinhoven P, et al. A meta-analysis of the treatment of panic disorder with or without agoraphobia: a comparison of psychopharmacological, cognitive-behavioural, and combination treatments. *J Nerv Ment Dis* 1997; **185**: 510–16.

35) d.
Functional behaviour assessment includes an account of the antecedents, the behaviour and the consequences; incubation is the increase in strength of conditioned response resulting from repeated brief exposure to the conditioned stimuli, and hence is important in ABC analysis.

36) b.
In alcohol dependency, aversion therapy is used; exposure and response prevention are mainly used to treat obsessive compulsive disorder.

37) d.
Punishment can effectively eliminate an undesirable response if it is consistent and is delivered immediately after the undesired response, and if an alternative response is rewarded. But when punishment fails to give an alternative response, the organism may substitute a less desirable response for the punished one.

38) b.

In systematic desensitization, patients attain a state of complete relaxation and are then exposed to the stimulus that elicits the anxiety response. The negative reaction of anxiety is inhibited by the relaxed state, a process called reciprocal inhibition. Systematic desensitization consists of three steps: relaxation training; hierarchy construction; and desensitization of the stimulus.

39) d.

Operant conditioning occurs only when the organism feels a contingency between its response and reinforcement, and hence is contingent on an anticipatory response.

40) d.

Magnification and minimization are cognitive distortions in depression. Fear of castration is the Freudian psychoanalytic theory that phobias represent a conflict, leading to avoidance of situations symbolic of that conflict.

41) d.

Over-inclusion (over-inclusive thinking) is a type of thinking described in schizophrenia where the patient is unable to preserve conceptual boundaries.

42) c.

Forgetting is different from extinction; in operant conditioning, a reinforcer is anything that increases the probability of a response when it follows the response (for example, food is reinforcing to a hungry animal; water is reinforcing to a thirsty animal; sex can be reinforcing to a sexually mature animal).

43) a.

The personality dimensions extroversion and neuroticism are normally distributed, whereas psychoticism is not.

44) d.

Kelly devised the Construct Repertory Test for eliciting a person's personal constructs.

45) c.

In Freud's structural model of the mind, small parts of the ego and superego are either in the conscious or in the preconscious.

46) e.

Non-directive psychotherapy is the same as client-centred therapy.

47) c.
A person whose self-schema includes being physically fit is more likely to exercise regularly.

48) b.
Sleepers who are awakened during NREM sleep report a dream about 50% of the time; sleepers who are awakened during REM sleep almost always report a dream.

49) c.
Older people tend to experience less stage 3 and 4 sleep.

50) e.
NREM sleep is associated with serotoninergic neuronal activity in the raphe complex; REM sleep is associated with noradrenergic neuronal activity.

51) d.
Sleep spindles and K complexes occur in stage 2 sleep.

Further reading

Puri B, Hall A. Chapters 1–3. In: *Revision Notes in Psychiatry*, 2nd edn. London: Arnold/Hodder Education, 2004.
Smith EE, Bem DJ, Nolen-Hoeksema S. Chapters 6–8. In: *Atkinson and Hilgard's Introduction to Psychology*, 14th edn. Florence, KY: Wadsworth Publishing Company, 2003.
Wright P, Stern J, Phelan M. *Core Psychiatry*, 2nd edn. London: Saunders, 2005.

3. Human development: Questions

1) Infants:
   a. By 3 months can recognize photographs of their mothers and prefer pictures of them to pictures of strangers
   b. By 5 months can remember faces of strangers
   c. Appear to be born with perceptual mechanisms that are already tuned to the properties of human speech
   d. Can discriminate among tastes and among odours soon after birth
   e. All of the above

2) All of the following are true about newborns' preferences for sounds, except:
   a. They prefer speech sounds over instrumental music
   b. They prefer heartbeats over male voices
   c. They prefer female voices over male voices
   d. They prefer their mother's voice to other women's voices
   e. They prefer their father's voice to other men's voices

3) Which age group is correctly paired with Piaget's stage of cognitive development?
   a. Birth to 2 years–Sensorimotor
   b. 2 to 5 years–Preoperational
   c. 5 to 9 years–Concrete operational
   d. 9 years and over–Formal operational
   e. All of the above

4) All of the following are true about Piaget's stages of cognitive development, except:
   a. Object permanence is achieved at the sensorimotor stage
   b. Egocentrism is characteristic of the preoperational stage
   c. Authoritarian morality is achieved in the concrete operational stage
   d. Laws of conservation and reversibility are achieved in the concrete operational stage
   e. In the formal operational stage, children can test a hypothesis systematically.

5) All of the following are characteristic of Piaget's preoperational stage, except:
   a. Animistic thinking
   b. Creationism
   c. Phenomenalistic causality and syncretism
   d. Precausal reasoning
   e. Symbolization

6) All of the following are behavioural dimensions identified by Thomas and Chess (1977) in infants, except:

  a. Activity level
  b. Rhythmicity
  c. Quality of mood
  d. Attention span and persistence
  e. Insecure attachment

7) All of the following attachment theorists' names are correctly paired with their observations, except:

  a. Harry Harlow—Social learning and the effects of social isolation in surrogate-reared monkeys
  b. John Bowlby—Attachment behaviour
  c. Mary Ainsworth—Transitional object
  d. Rene Spitz—Developmental retardation accompanies maternal rejection and neglect
  e. Margaret Mahler—Separation individualization

8) Regarding attachment in infants, which of the following statements is true?

  a. Monotropic attachment (to one individual) is less common than polytropic attachment
  b. Attachment usually takes place from mother to infant
  c. The attachment process can start soon after birth
  d. The attachment process takes an average of 3 months to complete
  e. Imprinting commonly occurs in primates

9) Attachment behaviours:

  a. Start to occur at the age of 6 months
  b. Are signs of distress shown by the child when separated from his/her attachment figure
  c. Include being more playful and talkative in the presence of the attachment figure
  d. Decrease visibly by 3 years
  e. All of the above

10) Insecure attachment:

  a. Is chronic clinginess and ambivalence towards the mother
  b. May be a precursor to childhood emotional disorders
  c. May be a precursor to school refusal
  d. May be a precursor to agoraphobia starting in adolescence
  e. All of the above

11) Regarding abnormalities in attachment:

a. Avoidant attachment caused by rejection by the mother may be a precursor to poor social functioning and aggression in later life
b. The rate of disappearance of separation anxiety varies with the child's temperament
c. Acute separation reaction described by Bowlby includes stages of protest, despair and detachment
d. Maternal deprivation can lead to developmental language delay
e. All of the above

12) Stranger anxiety:

a. Is shown by infants usually between the ages of 8 months and 1 year
b. Is identical to separation anxiety
c. Is more likely to appear in babies exposed to a variety of caretakers
d. Does not occur when the infant is in the mother's arms
e. All of the above

13) The theory of separation individualization proposed by Margaret Mahler includes all of the following, except:

a. Periods of sleep outweigh periods of arousal in the stage of normal autism between birth and 2 months
b. Mother–infant is perceived as a single fused entity in the symbiosis stage between 2 and 5 months
c. The infant starts to draw attention away from self to the outer world in the stage of practising between 10 and 18 months
d. Children move away from their mothers and come back for reassurance in the stage of rapprochement between 18 and 24 months
e. Children are reassured by the permanence of their mother in the stage of object constancy between 2 and 5 years of age

14) Regarding stages of development, all of the following are true, except:

a. If a child goes through the first 7 years without adequate vision, extensive permanent disability will result
b. Children who have not had enough exposure to language before age 6 or 7 may fail to acquire it all together
c. Although infants love to explore the faces of those who care for them, research has shown that they are attached not to the faces *per se* but to characteristics such as curved lines and movement complexity
d. A newborn can indicate a preference for certain sounds
e. According to Piaget, the process of a child's modifying the existing schema, to extend his/her theory of the world, is called assimilation

15) Failure to develop adequate attachments due to prolonged maternal separation can result in all of the following, except:

  a. An indiscriminate relationship with strangers in later childhood
  b. Development of obsessive compulsive disorder in early adulthood
  c. Attention seeking and over-activity at school
  d. Enuresis in later childhood
  e. Growth retardation

16) According to Piaget's stage theory:

  a. If a cloth is placed over a toy that an 8-month-old is reaching for, the infant immediately stops reaching and appears to lose interest in the toy
  b. 3–4-year-olds cannot think in symbolic terms, as their words and images are not yet organized in a logical manner
  c. Preoperational children are aware of perspectives other than their own
  d. Concrete operational thinking is dominated by visual impressions
  e. Adolescent thinking is characterized by egocentrism

17) At the age of 2 years normal children:

  a. Can refer to self by name and use pronouns
  b. Can express emotions like guilt and envy
  c. Can build a tower of nine or ten cubes
  d. Can copy a circle and a cross
  e. Can use language to describe incidents from the past

18) All of the following are associated with slower speech development, except:

  a. Bilingual home
  b. Larger family size
  c. Intrauterine growth retardation
  d. Prolonged second-stage labour
  e. Being a twin

19) Regarding temperament, all of the following are true, except:

  a. The nine categories identified by Thomas and Chess have been found to cluster as easy child (40%), difficult child (15%) and slow-to-warm-up child (10%)
  b. Some temperamental traits do not persist over time
  c. According to Bates, the neural basis of temperament emerges from the limbic system and the motor cortex
  d. Concepts of temperament can be useful in helping people solve problems
  e. In a study Capsi and Silva showed inhibited children at the age of 3 scored high on measures of impulsivity, danger seeking, aggression, and subsequent interpersonal alienation at the age of 18

20) Regarding moral development in children, Kohlberg's stage theory states that:

   a. In the pre-conventional stage up to the age of 7, morality is mainly reward and punishment oriented
   b. In the conventional stage (7–13), rules are conformed to in order to avoid the disapproval of others
   c. In the conventional stage, laws and social rules are upheld in order to avoid the censure of authorities
   d. The stage of post-conventional morality with social contract and ethical principle orientation may never be reached even in adulthood
   e. All of the above

21) Regarding social learning theory and sex typing, all of the following are true, except:

   a. Research suggests that human males are more physically aggressive than human females
   b. Observational learning enables children to imitate same-sex adults and thereby acquire sex-typed behaviours
   c. If a culture becomes less sex typed in ideology, children become less sex typed in their behaviour
   d. Fathers appear to be more concerned with sex-typed behaviour than mothers are, particularly with their sons
   e. Most 6- and 7-year-olds believe that there should be no sex-based restrictions on occupations

22) Regarding social learning theory and modelling, all of the following are true, except:

   a. Aggression in children may be learned by modelling
   b. Modelling has been shown to reduce anxiety
   c. Modelling was found to have no aetiological association with the development of personality disorders
   d. Fearful children become less fearful when they watch other children acting fearlessly in the same situation
   e. It is possible to eliminate negative behaviour patterns by having a person learn alternative techniques from other role models

23) Bandura:

   a. Regarded reinforcement and motivational processes as components of observational learning
   b. Proposed the concept of reciprocal determinism
   c. Observed that, in modelling, attention is attracted by models because of their distinctiveness, success, power and prestige
   d. Observed that people's choices of model are influenced by age, sex and similarity
   e. All of the above

24) Erik Erikson suggested that:
a. During child development there is a trust-versus-mistrust crisis between 3 and 5 years of age
b. At about 1−3 years, parental over-control or children's loss of self-control will result in muscular and anal impotence and produce a sense of doubt and shame
c. Between 3 and 5 years of age, excessive punishment leads to the development of a too-strong superego, but with a sense of responsibility, dependability and self-discipline
d. Between the ages of 6 and 11, if the parents reward children's industriousness at home, a school environment that denigrates or discourages children cannot diminish their self-esteem
e. If an identity crisis occurs at the end of adolescence it is abnormal

25) All of the following are related to Winnicott's theory, except:
a. True self
b. Holding environment
c. Good-enough mother
d. Transitional object
e. Paranoid-schizoid position

26) All of the following are true statements about Melanie Klein's work, except:
a. She viewed projection and repression as the primary defensive operations in the first months of life
b. She described a phenomenon of persecutory anxiety, when infants project derivatives of the death instinct onto the mother, and then fear attack from a 'bad mother'
c. The paranoid-schizoid position is characterized by the predominance of defence mechanism denial, splitting and primitive projective identification
d. In the depressive position, the mother is viewed ambivalently as having both positive and negative aspects
e. She developed a play technique in the psychoanalysis of children

27) Regarding the oral stage of Freud's stages of psychosexual development, all of the following are true, except:
a. It happens in approximately the first 18 months of life
b. Oral drives consist of two separate components: aggressive and libidinal
c. The aggressive components are thought to predominate in the early parts of the oral phase, whereas they are mixed with more libidinal components later
d. Excessive oral gratification or deprivation can result in libidinal fixations, leading to excessive optimism, narcissism and pessimism
e. Successful resolution of the oral phase provides a capacity to rely on others with a sense of trust and sense of self-reliance

28) Regarding the anal stage of Freud's stages of psychosexual development, all of the following are true, except:

a. It extends roughly from 1 to 5 years
b. Anal eroticism refers to the sexual pleasure in anal retention of faeces and in presenting them as a precious gift to parents
c. Anal sadism refers to the expression of aggressive wishes connected with discharging faeces as a powerful and destructive weapon
d. Anal characteristics and defences are most typically seen in obsessive compulsive neuroses
e. The urethral stage was treated by Freud as a transitional stage between anal and genital and the resolution of urethral conflicts sets the stage for budding gender identity

29) In the phallic stage of Freud's stages of psychosexual development:

a. The penis becomes the organ of principal interest in both sexes
b. The lack of a penis in the female is considered as evidence of castration
c. Castration anxiety arises in connection with guilt over masturbation and oedipal wishes
d. The influences of castration anxiety and penis envy, the defences against both, and the patterns of identification that emerge from the phallic phase are the primary determinants of the development of human character
e. Fixations and conflicts that derive from the preceding stages cannot usually modify the oedipal resolution

30) The concepts associated with Jungian theory are:

a. Collective unconsciousness
b. Archetypes and complexes
c. Introverts and extroverts
d. Individualization
e. All of the above

31) All of the following statements are correct, except:

a. Adler coined the term inferiority complex
b. Oral frustration and oral envy are terms used by Melanie Klein
c. Concepts associated with Winnicott include potential space and primary maternal preoccupation
d. Bion described the concept of basic assumptions
e. The concepts of 'container' and 'contained' and 'squiggle game' are associated with Anna Freud

32) Regarding family factors in child development, which of the following is true?

a. Vulnerability to unstable homes is influenced by sex and girls are more affected than boys
b. Vulnerability to unstable homes is influenced by age and older children are more vulnerable than younger children
c. In childhood and adolescence, the death of a parent is associated with adverse effects, such as an increase in later emotional problems, particularly a susceptibility to depression and divorce
d. Evidence indicates that working mothers raise children who are less healthy than those brought up by mothers who stay at home
e. When home caretakers act as surrogate mothers, children usually become more attached to the caretaker than to the parent

33) Regarding family factors in child development, all of the following statements are true, except:

a. Single parenting has been found to have an association with increased emotional and behavioural problems in children
b. Having two lesbian parents has been found to have an association with increased emotional and behavioural problems in children
c. Large family size has been found to have an association with increased emotional and behavioural problems in children
d. In dysfunctional families, marital conflicts may cause the parents to use a child with problems as a scapegoat
e. Parental divorce is associated with an increased rate of disturbance in children, greater than following parental bereavement

34) Death of a parent leads to:

a. Increased functional enuresis and increased temper tantrums in young children
b. Increased sleep disturbance in older children
c. Depressive reactions in girls
d. Impaired school performance
e. All of the above

35) All of the following statements about family functioning and parenting are true, except:

a. An association has been established between child psychiatric disorders and exposure to family discord
b. Rutter described four patterns of family interaction: enmeshment, overprotection, rigidity and lack of conflict resolution
c. Authoritative parenting leads to good peer and parental relationships
d. With authoritarian parenting, boys may be more aggressive and girls less motivated
e. With indulgent parenting, children are often positive but can be immature and the lack of authority may lead to increased aggressive behaviour

36) All of the following are recognized sequelae of sexual abuse in children, except:

a. Eating disorders
b. Depression
c. Paranoid reactions and mistrust
d. Neurological impairment
e. Borderline personality disorder

37) All of the following are recognized sequelae of physical abuse in children, except:

a. Depression
b. Dissociation
c. Borderline personality disorder
d. Delayed language development
e. Eating disorder

38) All of the following statements about development of fears in childhood are true, except:

a. Fear of novel stimuli begins at 6 months, reaching a peak at 1 year
b. Fear of heights begins at 6–8 months
c. In the preschool age group, the common fears are of animals, the dark and monsters
d. Fear of shameful social situations begins between 6 and 11 years of age
e. Fears of death, failure and social gatherings dominate in adolescence

39) All of the following statements about fears and dreams in childhood are true, except:

a. Freud proposed that displacement of fear of castration to situations symbolic of that conflict leads to development of phobias
b. Most 3-year-olds understand that dreams are unique to each individual
c. Newborns were found to have some brain activity similar to that of the dreaming state
d. At the age of 5–6, dreams of being killed or injured and of ghosts become prominent
e. Adults spend 20% of sleeping time dreaming

40) All of the following statements about sexual development are true, except:

a. Over-ripeness of the ovum at fertilization is associated with a masculinizing effect on genetic females
b. In 80% of girls the onset of puberty is marked by pubic hair growth
c. Between ages 17 and 18 luteinizing hormone is frequently elevated above adult values
d. In adolescent boys, testosterone levels correlate with libido and are manifested by sex drive and masturbation
e. An increase in suprarenal androgen release (adrenarche) usually begins between the ages of 6 and 8

41) Regarding gender identity and sexual orientation, all of the following are true, except:

    a. Gender identity is usually established by the age of 3 or 4 years and usually remains firmly established thereafter

    b. Sexual drive exists from birth to middle childhood and increases again during adolescence

    c. Sexual fantasy is the most important dimension in assessing homosexual orientation

    d. Research has shown that childhood gender non-conformity is a strong indicator of genetic loading for homosexuality

    e. In pedigree and linkage analyses of homosexual men, increased rates of homosexual orientation were found in the maternal uncles and male cousins, but not in their fathers or paternal relatives

42) All of the following include the adolescent identity statuses suggested by Marcia, except:

    a. Adolescent turmoil

    b. Identity achievement

    c. Foreclosure

    d. Moratorium

    e. Identity diffusion

43) The symptomatology of normal grief does not include:

    a. A feeling of numbness as a result of initial shock and disbelief and denial of anger

    b. Adopting the mannerisms and characteristics of the deceased person (identification phenomena)

    c. Somatic symptoms, including biological symptoms of depression

    d. Intense anger and feelings of betrayal persisting up to 6 months after bereavement

    e. Misery and searching behaviour persisting for up to 6 months after bereavement

44) About the grief reaction, all of the following are true, except:

    a. The initial stages of grief described by Parks include alarm and numbness

    b. In the stage of pining described by Parks, illusions or hallucinations of the deceased may occur

    c. In the depressive stage of grief described by Parks, disorganization and despair occur

    d. If a parent/caregiver dies before the development of attachment behaviour, grief reaction is still seen in babies

    e. Grief reactions of any duration, considered to be abnormal because of their form or content, are classified under adjustment disorders in ICD-10

45) According to Erikson:

a. Initiative versus guilt is the dominant theme between 3 and 5 years
b. Intimacy versus isolation dominates in adolescence
c. Industry versus inferiority dominates in early adulthood
d. Generativity versus stagnation is the dominant theme after 65 years of age
e. All of the above are true

46) Regarding intelligence tests, all of the following are true, except:

a. The most recent revision of the Stanford–Binet Intelligence Scale uses IQ scores instead of standard age scores
b. The 1986 revised Stanford–Binet Intelligence Scale tests four broad areas: verbal reasoning; abstract/visual reasoning; quantitative reasoning; and short-term memory
c. The Wechsler Adult Intelligence Scale is divided into two parts (a verbal and a performance scale) that yield separate scores as well as a full-scale IQ
d. The Scholastic Assessment Test and the American College Test are examples of group-administered general ability tests
e. According to Spearman's factor analysis, the g factor is the major determinant of performance on intelligence tests and the s factor is specific to particular abilities or tests

47) Regarding contemporary theories of intelligence, which of the following names is correctly paired with the theory?

a. Howard Gardner–Theory of multiple intelligences
b. Mike Anderson–Theory of intelligence and cognitive development
c. Robert Sternberg–Triarchic theory
d. Stephen Ceci–Bioecological theory
e. All of the above

48) Regarding assessment of personality, all of the following are true, except:

a. When Cattell's 16 factors are factor analysed, Eysenck's two factors emerge as super-factors
b. Most personality tests ask individuals to directly rate themselves on personality trait dimensions
c. The Minnesota Multiphasic Personality Inventory (MMPI) is less successful in making finer distinctions among various forms of psychopathology
d. The MMPI is widely used to study normal populations
e. Q-sort is a special method of measuring personality traits, in which a rater or sorter describes an individual's personality by sorting a set of approximately 100 cards into piles

49) All of the following are true about the psychoanalytic approach to personality, except:

   a. The superego develops in response to parental rewards and punishments
   b. Aggressive impulses may be expressed in disguised form by racing sports cars, playing chess, or making sarcastic remarks
   c. A projective test presents an ambiguous stimulus to which the person may respond as he/she wishes
   d. The Rorschach test is usually done in two phases, the first being a free-association phase and the second an inquiry phase
   e. The Thematic Apperception Test is more useful as a basis for making a diagnosis than as a technique for inferring motivational aspects of behaviour

50) All of the following are true about personality theories, except:

   a. According to Kelly, personal constructs take an either/or form
   b. Kelly's Construct Repertory Test technique is useful for counselling
   c. Bannister's repertory grid can be used to measure formal thought disorder
   d. Most individuals conform to Kretschmer's three personality categories linked to body build as pyknic, asthenic and athletic
   e. Rogers proposed that a large discrepancy between ideal self and real self results in an unhappy, dissatisfied person

3. Human development: Answers

1) e.
There are sensitive periods optimal for a particular type of development. If cataracts are removed before the age of 7, vision will develop fairly normally. The first year of life appears to be a sensitive period for the formation of interpersonal attachments. The preschool period is sensitive for intellectual and language acquisition.

2) e.
A newborn can indicate a preference for certain sounds by sucking more vigorously on a nipple when preferred sounds are played through an earphone.

3) a.
Preoperational, 2 to 7 years; concrete operational, 7 to 11 years; formal operational, 11 years and over.

4) c.
Authoritarian morality is achieved in the preoperational stage.

5) e.
Symbolization expressed in mental symbols and words occurs in the sensor motor stage. Animism attributes life and feelings to inanimate objects. Phenomenalistic causality claims that events that occur together are thought to cause one another.

6) e.
The nine behavioural dimensions identified by Thomas and Chess include approach or withdrawal, adaptability, intensity of reaction, threshold of responsiveness, and distractibility, in addition to a, b, c and d.

Thomas A, Chess S. *Temperament and Development*. New York: Brunner/ Mazel, 1977.

7) c.
Ainsworth, expanding on Bowlby's observations, confirmed that attachment serves the purpose of reducing anxiety and observed that inanimate objects also serve as a secure base; however, Donald Winnicott called these inanimate objects transitional objects.

8) c.
Monotropic attachment (to one individual, usually the mother) is more common than polytropic attachment. Attachment usually takes place from infant to mother and neonatal–maternal bonding takes place in the opposite direction. The attachment process takes an average of 6 months

to complete. Imprinting described by Lorenz is the phenomenon of geese following the first nearby moving object soon after hatching, and there is no evidence that this occurs in primates.

9) e.
Attachment behaviour is an infant's tendency to seek closeness to particular people and to feel more secure in their presence.

10) e.
Insecure attachment can be avoidant or ambivalent.

11) e.
Studies suggest that children who are securely attached by the time they enter their second year are better equipped to cope with new experiences.

12) a.
Separation anxiety occurs between 10 and 18 months of age; it is related to stranger anxiety but not identical to it.

13) c.
An infant starts to draw attention away from self to the outer world in the stage of differentiation (between 5 and 10 months), and the ability to move autonomously increases in the stage of practising (between 10 and 18 months).

14) c.
According to Piaget, a child understanding a novel object or event, in terms of a pre-existing schema, is an example of assimilation; the process of the child's modifying the existing schema, to extend his/her theory of the world, is called accommodation.

15) b.
In psychoanalysis, the origin of obsessional personality is located at the anal stage of development.

16) a.
3–4-year-olds can think in symbolic terms, and by about 18 months to 2 years they start using symbols. Preoperational thinking is characterized by egocentrism, when children are unaware of perspectives other than their own, and this stage is dominated by visual impressions. In the concrete operational stage they start using abstract thinking and reach formal operations by the age of 11 or 12.

17) a.
Emotional expression develops as follows: tender affection and shame at 12–18 months; pride at 2 years; guilt and shame at 3–4 years. Motor and behavioural development happens as follows: at 2 years a child can go up and down stairs alone, build a tower of six or seven cubes, and parallel play; at 3 years a child can build towers of nine or ten cubes, copy a circle and a cross, and feed itself well; at 4 years a child can use language to describe incidents from the past.

18) a.
Having a bilingual home is not a disadvantage. Female sex, being middle class, etc. are associated with faster, early language development.

19) e.
In a study Caspi and Silva showed uncontrolled children at the age of 3 scored high on measures of impulsivity, danger seeking, aggression, and subsequent interpersonal alienation at the age of 18, and inhibited children scored low.

Caspi A, Silva P. Temperamental qualities at age 3 predict personality traits in young adulthood: Longitudinal evidence from a birth cohort. *Child Dev* 1995; **66**: 486–98.

20) e.
Kohlberg described six developmental stages of moral judgement categorized into three levels. Pre-conventional morality is level 1 and the stages here include stage 1 (punishment orientation) and stage 2 (reward orientation). Conventional morality is level 2 and the stages are stage 3 (good boy/good girl orientation) and stage 4 (authority orientation). Level 3 is post-conventional morality and stages here are stage 5 (social contract orientation) and stage 6 (ethical principle orientation).

21) e.
Most 6- and 7-year-olds believe that there should be sex-based restrictions on occupations, as they hold more rigid opinions (Piaget's preoperational) but 4-year-olds and 9-year-olds believe that there should be no sex-based restrictions on occupations.

22) c.
In modelling, the person learns behaviours by observing others and it is thought to be linked to the development of personality disorders, since maladaptive behaviours can be learnt through modelling.

23) e.
Bandura promotes the behaviourist/social learning approach. Bandura suggested four components to observational learning: attentional process; retention process; motor reproduction process; and reinforcement and motivational processes.

24) b.

Erikson's stages of life cycle are as follows: stage 1 (birth to 1 year), trust versus mistrust is the first crisis and towards the second half of the first year an oral crisis occurs; stage 2 (1−3 years), autonomy versus shame and doubt; stage 3 (3−5 years), excessive punishment can restrict children's imagination and development of a too-strong superego may become dangerous for themselves and others; stage 4 (6−11 years), industry versus inferiority; stage 5 (from 11 years to adolescence), identity versus role diffusion and identity crisis is regarded as normal; stage 6 (21−40 years), intimacy versus self-absorption; stage 7 (40−65 years), generativity versus stagnation; stage 8 (over 65 years), integrity versus despair and isolation.

25) e.

The paranoid-schizoid position is described by Melanie Klein. Winnicott is a central figure in the British school of object relations theory. He developed the theory of multiple self-organizations.

26) a.

Melanie Klein viewed projection and introjection as the primary defensive operations in the first months of life.

27) c.

The libidinal components are thought to predominate in the early parts of the oral phase (oral erotism), whereas they are mixed with more aggressive components later (oral sadism).

28) a.

The anal stage of Freud's stages of psychosexual development extends roughly from 1 to 3 years.

29) e.

Fixations and conflicts deriving from the preceding stages can contaminate and modify the oedipal resolution.

30) e.

Collective unconsciousness (objective psyche) contains latent memories of our cultural, racial and phylogenetic past. Jung theory employs causality, teleology and synchronicity. Archetypes include anima, animus, persona, shadow and self. Jung identified four mental operations: feeling, intuition, sensation and thinking.

31) e.

The concepts of 'container' and 'contained' are associated with Wilfred Bion, and the 'squiggle game' with Winnicott.

32) c.
Regarding vulnerability to unstable homes, boys are more affected than girls, and older children are less vulnerable than younger ones.

33) b.
Having two lesbian parents was not identified as a harmful factor.

34) e.
Increased temper tantrums and prolonged bereavement reactions occur.

35) b.
Minuchin described four patterns of family interaction and Rutter described four types of parenting styles: authoritarian (leading to childhood depression); permissive (leading to poor impulse control in children); indifferent (leading to aggressive behaviour in children); and reciprocal (leading to a sense of self-reliance in children).

36) d.
Post-traumatic stress disorder (PTSD) and increased drug and alcohol abuse also occur.

37) e.
Neurological impairment is associated with physical abuse, whereas eating disorders are associated with sexual abuse.

38) a.
Fear of novel stimuli begins at 6 months, reaching a peak at 18 months to 2 years.

39) b.
At the age of 3 years, many children believe that dreams are directly shared by more than one person, but most 4-year-olds understand that dreams are unique to each individual.

40) b.
In 80% of girls the onset of puberty is marked by breast formation and in 20% by pubic hair growth.

41) d.
In a study Bailey and Pillard found that childhood gender non-conformity did not appear to be an indicator of genetic loading for homosexuality.

Bailey JM, Pillard RC. A genetic study of male sexual orientation. *Arch Gen Psychiatry* 1991; **48**: 1089–96.

42) a.

Affective stability and adolescent turmoil were described by Anna Freud, Erikson, and Offer and Offer.

Puri B, Hall A. Chapter 5. In: *Revision Notes in Psychiatry*, 2nd edn. London: Arnold/Hodder Education, 2004.
Wright P, Stern J, Phelan M. Chapter 4. In: *Core Psychiatry*, 2nd edn. London: Saunders, 2005.

43) d.

Intense anger and feelings of betrayal persisting beyond 6 weeks after bereavement are regarded as an abnormal grief reaction.

44) d.

If a parent/caregiver dies before the development of attachment behaviour, grief reaction is not seen in babies.

45) a.

Erikson's stages of life cycle are as follows: stage 1 (birth to 1 year), trust versus mistrust is the first crisis and towards the second half of the first year an oral crisis occurs; stage 2 (1–3 years), autonomy versus shame and doubt; stage 3 (3–5 years), excessive punishment can restrict children's imagination and development of a too-strong superego may become dangerous for themselves and others; stage 4 (6–11 years), industry versus inferiority; stage 5 (from 11 years to adolescence), identity versus role diffusion and identity crisis is regarded as normal; stage 6 (21–40 years), intimacy versus self-absorption; stage 7 (40–65 years), generativity versus stagnation; stage 8 (over 65 years), integrity versus despair and isolation.

46) a.

The most recent revision of the Stanford–Binet Intelligence Scale uses standard age scores instead of IQ scores.

47) e.

Gardner identified seven distinct kinds of intelligence that are independent of one another: linguistic intelligence; logical-mathematical intelligence; musical intelligence; bodily-kinaesthetic intelligence; spatial intelligence; interpersonal intelligence; and intrapersonal intelligence.

48) b.

Most personality tests do not actually ask individuals to directly rate themselves on personality trait dimensions; instead they are asked a set of questions about how they react in certain situations. Using factor analysis, Cattell in his trait theory derived 16 personality factors. Using second-order factor analysis, three broad dimensions were identified: sociability (extra/intra), anxiety and intelligence. Eysenck had a dimensional approach, and using factor analysis he described orthogonal dimensions, which were assumed to be normally distributed. These include neuroticism/stability, extroversion/introversion, psychoticism/stability, and intelligence. Personality inventories used to measure these traits are the MPI (Maudsley Personality Inventory), EPI (Eysenck Personality Inventory) and EPQ (Eysenck Personality Questionnaire). The Minnesota Multiphasic Personality Inventory (MMPI) consists of lengthy, true/false/cannot say answers and is empirically constructed and widely used. It measures traits.

Puri B, Hall A. Chapter 33. In: *Revision Notes in Psychiatry*, 2nd edn. London: Arnold/Hodder Education, 2004.

49) e.
The Thematic Apperception Test is more useful as a technique for inferring motivational aspects of behaviour than as a basis for making a diagnosis. The Rorschach ink blot test is a projective test.

50) d.
Kretschmer used, a categorical approach, which is widely used, but most people do not conform to categories.

Further reading

Puri B, Hall A. Chapters 5–6. In: *Revision Notes in Psychiatry*, 2nd edn. London: Arnold/Hodder Education, 2004.
Sadock BJ, Sadock VA. Chapters 2–6. In: *Kaplan and Sadock's Synopsis of Psychiatry*, 10th edn. Baltimore, MD: Lippincott, Williams and Wilkins, 2008.
Smith EE, Bem DJ, Nolen-Hoeksema S. Chapters 2–3. In: *Atkinson and Hilgard's Introduction to Psychology*, 14th edn. Florence, KY: Wadsworth Publishing Company, 2003.
Wright P, Stern J, Phelan M. *Core Psychiatry*, 2nd edn. London: Saunders, 2005.

4. Social psychology and basic psychological treatments: Questions

Social psychology and social sciences

1) Attitudes:
   a. Are a set of beliefs which predispose an individual to particular ideas
   b. Have affective components that are most resistant to change
   c. Are mutually consistent and internally consistent
   d. If situational variables are not taken into account, measured attitudes are poor predictors of behaviour
   e. All of the above

2) In measurements of attitudes:
   a. Projective tests such as Rorschach ink blots are useful
   b. Physiological tests such as galvanic skin response are useful
   c. More easily administered Likert scales and visual analogue scales like semantic differential scales are useful
   d. Thurstone scales are less sensitive than Likert scales and can have value-laden biases
   e. All of the above

3) The social effects that have an impact on measurements of behaviour are:
   a. Response set
   b. Bias to middle
   c. Halo effect
   d. Hawthorn effect
   e. All of the above

4) Regarding attitudes and behaviours, all of the following are true, except:
   a. Advertising uses a central pathway requiring the consideration of new information to modify one's attitude
   b. Advertising uses a peripheral pathway involving the presentation of cues to modify one's attitude
   c. The characteristics of a persuasive communicator include attractiveness and credibility
   d. Low self-esteem and intelligence of the recipient increase the likelihood that complex communications will be persuasive
   e. A low-anxiety recipient is more influenced by a high-fear message and vice versa

5) Regarding persuasive influence leading to attitude change, all of the following are true, except:

   a. Message repetition can be a persuasive influence leading to attitude change
   b. Implicit messages are more persuasive for more intelligent recipients
   c. One-sided communications are more persuasive for those who are less intelligent
   d. Mass media communication is more persuasive than interactive personal discussions
   e. Social change is sometimes brought about because a few people manage to persuade the majority to change attitudes

6) According to Festinger's cognitive dissonance theory, dissonance is increased by all of the following, except:

   a. Low pressure to comply
   b. Increased choice of options
   c. Adding new cognitions
   d. Awareness of responsibility for consequences
   e. Expectation of unpleasant consequences of behaviour towards others

7) All of the following names are correctly paired with the appropriate concept, except:

   a. Carl Rogers—Self-actualization and self-direction
   b. Daryl Bem—Self-perception theory
   c. Leon Festinger—Social exchange theory
   d. Fritz Heider—Attribution theory
   e. Theodore Newcomb—Reinforcement theory

8) Regarding social facilitation and social inhibition, all of the following are true, except:

   a. Studies show that people performed better on the Stroop task when in the presence of others
   b. Audience effects on performance vary depending on whether the task is very easy or difficult for the person and on how much the person feels that he/she is being evaluated
   c. People often behave differently in a crowd than when alone, and they may experience de-individualization
   d. Research shows that people are more likely to help a man lying on the sidewalk if many other bystanders are present
   e. Modern warfare allows individuals to distance themselves from actual killing, giving them the feeling that they are not responsible for enemy deaths

9) All of the following statements about factors relating to interpersonal attraction are true, except:

   a. Neighbours are likely to form a friendship simply because of proximity
   b. People prefer relationships that appear to have an optimum cost:benefit ratio
   c. Complimentarity is more important than similarity, although the latter increases in importance with time
   d. Partners in successful long-term relationships tend to be similar to each other in characteristics such as age, race, education and physical attractiveness
   e. In later life, the passionate component of romantic love tends to become less important than the companionate component

10) All of the following are true about theories relating to interpersonal issues and intergroup behaviour, except:

   a. According to Heider's attribution theory, internal (dispositional) attribution is the inference that the person is primarily responsible for the action
   b. Primary attribution error is a bias towards situational rather than dispositional attribution when inferring the cause of other people's behaviour
   c. Stereotypes persist even if data do not confirm them
   d. Stereotypes can become self-perpetuating and self-fulfilling
   e. Prejudiced individuals may behave in ways that create stereotyped behaviour, which sustain their prejudice

11) All of the following are true about observations related to social influence, except:

   a. Autocratic leadership is useful in urgent situations
   b. Democratic leadership yields greater productivity
   c. Laissez-faire is appropriate for creative and person-oriented tasks
   d. Audience effect is the social facilitation occurring when others simply observe
   e. Intelligent, expressive and socially effective individuals are most vulnerable to group pressure

12) All of the following are true about theories of social influence, except:

   a. French and Raven observed that social power could be derived from skill, knowledge, experience and power to punish
   b. Normative social influence can lead to an individual's agreeing with a group even if the individual holds a different personal view
   c. Conformity pressures increase with group size up to a maximum of three
   d. Milgram demonstrated that obedience is affected by proximity to the victim, with decreased obedience with distance
   e. Informational social influence is more evident with ambiguous stimuli

13) All of the following are true about groupthink, except:

    a. It may include collective rationalization and 'mindguards'

    b. It may lead to decisions that are based on incomplete information

    c. It is helpful in preventing decisions that have failed to fully examine all the risks and consider alternative plans

    d. It can be guarded against by having open debates

    e. It can be guarded against by appointing a 'devil's advocate' or using external experts

14) All of the following disorders are more likely to be diagnosed in lower social classes, except:

    a. Alcohol dependence

    b. Personality disorder

    c. Bipolar disorder

    d. Schizophrenia

    e. Organic psychosis

15) Regarding social, family factors in relation to illnesses, all of the following names are correctly paired with their related concept, except:

    a. Parsons—Sick role

    b. Mechanic—Illness behaviour

    c. Fromm-Reichman—Schizophrenogenic mother

    d. Bateson—Double bind

    e. Vaughn and Leff—Marital skew and marital schism

16) Regarding effects of expressed emotion, all of the following statements are true, except:

    a. Comments expressing unambiguous dislike or disapproval are associated with high expressed emotion and predict relapse of schizophrenia

    b. Emotional over-involvement is associated with high expressed emotion and predict relapse of schizophrenia

    c. Positive remarks expressing praise or approval of the patient are not associated with high expressed emotion

    d. Follow-up studies have confirmed that, in the presence of high expressed emotion in the family, the relapse rates of treated and untreated patients with schizophrenia are almost the same

    e. High expressed emotion at home is associated with an increased risk of relapse of depression

17) The four vulnerability factors identified by Brown and Harris that make women more susceptible to depression following life events do not include:

a. The loss of their mother before the age of 11 years
b. Not working outside the home
c. The lack of a confiding relationship
d. Problems with in-laws
e. Having three or more children under the age of 15 years at home

18) On the Holmes and Rahe social readjustment scale, which of the following life events was given the highest life change value?

a. Death of a spouse
b. Divorce
c. Marital separation
d. Jail term
e. Death of a close family member

19) Studies observed a clear relationship between life events and all of the following conditions, except:

a. Onset of depression
b. First onset of schizophrenia
c. Anxiety
d. Deliberate self-harm
e. Functional disorders presenting physically without an organic cause

20) Which of the following names is associated with studies related to the concept of institutionalization?

a. Goffman
b. Barton
c. Wing
d. Brown
e. All of the above

Basic psychological treatments

21) A 45-year-old man was clearly told about the bad prognosis of his wife's cancer in the previous outpatient appointment a month ago, but he tells you that he does not have any memory of that conversation. The possible defence mechanism involved is:

a. Repression
b. Denial
c. Projection
d. Displacement
e. Regression

22) A 38-year-old man who had strong sexual fantasies towards another woman attributed his impulses and desires to his wife and became extremely jealous and possessive of her. The possible defence mechanism involved is:

a. Projection
b. Identification
c. Projective identification
d. Reaction formation
e. Displacement

23) A 23-year-old woman diagnosed with personality disorder walked out of the ward round room after becoming argumentative, and on her way out she kicked a chair in the corridor. The possible defence mechanism involved is:

a. Reaction formation
b. Displacement
c. Acting out
d. Turning against self
e. Identification with aggressor

24) On an assessment for psychotherapy it was formulated that a 24-year-old woman with obsessive compulsive disorder was secretly fascinated with urine; she started rejecting and denying all interest in urine and developed an obsessive need for cleaning her hands. The possible defence mechanism involved is:

a. Reaction formation
b. Magic undoing
c. Isolation
d. Intellectualization
e. Splitting

25) A 40-year-old man with obsessive compulsive disorder tells you that by touching lamp posts in a specific order he attempts to recreate the past so that he can avoid some horrible things he is worried about. If the particular order is missed he needs to start again from the beginning. The possible defence mechanism is:

a. Reaction formation
b. Magic undoing
c. Isolation
d. Intellectualization
e. Splitting

26) All of the following are true about psychoanalysis, except:

    a. The primary focus is on analyst and intrasession events
    b. It is transference-neurosis facilitated
    c. Regression is discouraged
    d. Symptom relief is an indirect result
    e. The free association method predominates

27) In an expressive form of psychotherapy, the therapist said to the patient, who was late, 'Perhaps the reason you are late is that you were afraid I would react the way your father reacted to the success you are now having.' The psychotherapeutic intervention used here is:

    a. Interpretation
    b. Confrontation
    c. Clarification
    d. Encouragement to elaborate
    e. Empathic validation

28) In Freud's interpretation of dreams, which of the following mechanisms was considered as facilitating the discharge of latent impulses?

    a. Condensation
    b. Displacement
    c. Symbolic representation
    d. Secondary revision
    e. All of the above

29) All the following names are correctly paired with the form of brief psychotherapy associated with their work, except:

    a. Brief focal psychotherapy–Balint and Malan
    b. Time-limited psychotherapy–Mann
    c. Interpersonal psychotherapy–Sullivan, Weissman and Klerman
    d. Dialectical therapy–Ryle
    e. Short-term dynamic psychotherapy–Davanloo

30) All of the following statements are correct regarding cognitive analytic therapy, except:

    a. It involves reformulation, the patient being helped to recognize the recurrences of unrevised patterns, and is open to revision
    b. It describes traps as negative assumptions that generate acts that produce consequences and reinforce assumptions
    c. It describes dilemmas as a person acting on false dichotomies, usually unaware that this is the case
    d. It describes snags as the abandonment of appropriate roles because of the assumption that others will oppose them
    e. It requires very well structured sessions with diagrams and homework until the end of the therapy

31) Transference:

a. Can assist treatment
b. May impede treatment
c. May lead to excessive dependency
d. May help patients to learn more about themselves
e. All of the above

32) Regarding small-group therapy, all of the following are true, except:

a. It can be used to modify personality problems
b. It has specific goals, i.e. high leader activity includes cognitive behavioural therapy carried out in a group setting
c. Yalom's curative factors in a group treatment include selective abstraction
d. Results are generally thought to be better with patients who are young, well motivated and free from personality disorder
e. Severe social anxiety is a contraindication

33) All of the following are contraindications to the therapeutic community method of treatment, except:

a. Severe depression
b. Hypomania
c. Dissocial personality disorder
d. Schizophrenia
e. Persistent violence

34) The principal features of a therapeutic community include all of the following, except:

a. Informality
b. Altruism
c. Permissiveness
d. Shared decisions
e. Shared activity

35) In cognitive psychotherapy, disattribution technique is most useful as an intervention to identify and correct the following cognitive error:

a. Overgeneralizing
b. Selective abstraction
c. Excessive responsibility
d. Catastrophizing
e. Dichotomous thinking

36) The key element of supportive therapy is:

a. The interview
b. Reassurance and explanation
c. Guidance and suggestion
d. Ventilation
e. All of the above

37) All of the following statements about functional analysis are true, except:

a. Problem clarification is an important component of functional analysis
b. Motivational analysis is an important component of functional analysis
c. Developmental analysis is an important component of functional analysis
d. Transactional analysis is an important component of functional analysis
e. Exploration of social relationships is an important component of functional analysis

38) The cognitive distortions in depression identified by Beck include all of the following, except:

a. Arbitrary inference
b. Selective abstraction
c. Ambivalence
d. Overgeneralization
e. Personalization

39) A 26-year-old woman with anxiety was given a prompt card by her therapist. On the card a reassuring thought was written: 'My heart is beating fast because I feel anxious, not because I have heart disease'. This is an example of which cognitive technique?

a. Distraction
b. Neutralizing
c. Challenging
d. Reassessing
e. Biofeedback

40) Social skills training was found to be helpful in:

a. Patients with incapacitating interpersonal issues
b. Depression
c. Agoraphobia
d. Rehabilitation in psychosis
e. All of the above

41) The following names are correctly paired with the form of therapy they have developed, except:

    a. Janov–Primal therapy
    b. Ellis–Rational emotive therapy
    c. Pearls–Gestalt therapy
    d. Berne–Psychodrama
    e. Frankl–Existential logotherapy

42) Couple therapy is not recommended in all the following scenarios, except:

    a. When there is conflict about one of the partner's sexual life
    b. When one of the partners suffers from a severe form of psychosis
    c. When one or both partners want to divorce
    d. When one spouse refuses to participate because of anxiety
    e. When one spouse refuses to participate because of fear

43) Which of the following is an example of a mature defence mechanism?

    a. Introjection
    b. Projective identification
    c. Intellectualization
    d. Rationalization
    e. Sublimation

44) All of the following are true about transference, except:

    a. It refers to the therapist's attitude towards the patient
    b. It is a repetition of reactions originating in regard to significant persons in early childhood
    c. It is inappropriate
    d. It occurs in non-therapeutic situations
    e. It could be an agent for therapeutic change

45) The characteristic regime in a therapeutic community as described by Rapoport includes:

    a. Permissiveness
    b. Reality confrontation
    c. Democracy
    d. Communalism
    e. All of the above

46) All of the following are true statements about psychoanalytic theory that explains obsessive symptoms, except:

a. Obsessional symptoms result from unconscious impulses of an aggressive nature
b. Obsessional symptoms result from unconscious impulses of a sexual nature
c. Anxiety is reduced by the action of defence mechanism of repression
d. Anxiety is reduced by the action of defence mechanism of reaction formation
e. Obsessional symptoms occur when there is a regression to the oral stage of development

47) All of the following defence mechanisms are paired with the condition associated with them, except:

a. Repression–Conversion disorder
b. Isolation–Obsessive compulsive disorder
c. Projection and splitting–Paranoia
d. Magical undoing–Depression
e. Displacement–Phobias

48) In the treatment of acute conversion disorder, it is recommended that:

a. Confrontation is almost always necessary to avoid reinforcement of disability and symptoms
b. A complete physical examination and investigation should not be attempted as it may reinforce the symptoms
c. Positive reassurance and praising healthy behaviour help to avoid reinforcement of disability and symptoms
d. The patient should not be provided with a face-saving opportunity as it may lead to reinforcement of disability and symptoms
e. All of the above

49) Regarding cognitive behaviour therapy, all of the following are true, except:

a. It is designed to change cognitions and behaviour directly
b. It is concerned with the way the disorder has developed
c. It focuses on the factors that are maintaining the disorder at the time of treatment
d. The patient is an active partner
e. Therapeutic procedures are usually presented as experiments

50) A 40-year-old woman who believes that she will faint during a panic attack tells you that she tenses her muscles every time she feels anxious, because she is convinced that she would have fainted had she not done this on every occasion. This is an example of:

a. Avoidance
b. Safety behaviour
c. Selective attention
d. Overgeneralization
e. Arbitrary inference

4. Social psychology and basic psychological treatments: Answers

1) e.
The definition of attitude was given by Allport as a mental and neural state of readiness, organized through experience, exerting an influence on an individual's response to all objects and situations. Kerch and Crutchfield defined the motivational, emotional, perceptual and cognitive components. Beliefs, behaviour and affective components were identified; a change in one of these three components leads to change in the others.

2) e.
The Thurstone scale is dichotomous, the Likert scale is generally a five-point scale of level of agreement and the semantic differential scale is a bipolar visual analogue scale.

3) e.
Response set is a tendency to always agree/disagree with a set of questions. Bias to middle is avoiding extreme response. The halo effect occurs when an observer allows a preconception to influence responses. The Hawthorn effect occurs when positive social interaction between the experimenter and the subject affects response.

4) d.
Advertising uses both a and b. Other characteristics of a persuasive communicator include audience identification with the communicator, being an opinion leader, non-verbal communication, and views of reference groups. High self-esteem and intelligence of the recipient increase the likelihood that complex communications will be persuasive.

5) d.
Mass media communication is less persuasive than interactive personal discussions.

6) c.
By adding new cognitions, dissonance is decreased. Dismissing information/cognitions and changing behaviour also result in a decrease in dissonance.

7) c.
Carl Rogers was associated with the person-centred theory of personality and psychotherapy, in which the major concepts are self-actualization and self-direction. He developed client-centred therapy. Bem's self-perception theory proposes that we make judgements about ourselves using the same inferential processes and errors that we use for making judgements about others. Festinger proposed social comparison theory and Homans proposed social exchange theory.

8) d.

Research shows that people are more likely to help a man lying on the sidewalk if no other bystanders are present.

9) c.

Similarity is more important than complimentarity, although the latter increases in importance with time.

10) b.

Primary attribution error is a bias towards dispositional rather than situational attribution when inferring the cause of other people's behaviour.

11) e.

Intelligent, expressive and socially effective individuals are least vulnerable to group pressure.

12) d.

Milgram demonstrated that obedience is affected by proximity to the victim, with increased obedience with distance. French and Raven described five types of social power: authority, reward, coercive, referent and expert. Deutsch and Gerard described two types of conformity: informational and normative.

13) c.

Groupthink is the desire to achieve consensus and avoid dissent in group decisions. Mindguards are individuals who are self-appointed to prevent the group from considering information that would challenge the effectiveness of the group. Groupthink leads to decisions that have failed to examine fully all the risks and to consider alternative plans.

14) c.

Depression in women and deliberate self-harm are also more likely to be diagnosed in lower social classes, whereas anorexia and bulimia in females are more likely to be diagnosed in upper classes.

15) e.

The concept of marital skew and marital schism was proposed by Lidz. Vaughn and Leff, and Brown are associated with expressed emotion and Wynne is associated with abnormal family communication.

16) d.

Vaughn and Leff observed that, in the presence of high expressed emotion, the relapse rate was higher in untreated patients than that in treated patients.

17) d.

High expressed emotion can be associated with relapse of depression.

18) a.
The highest life change value is for death of spouse, the values going from a to e in decreasing order.

19) b.
Brown, Birley and Tennant observed that independent life events are more likely to occur before relapse rather than before first onset of schizophrenia.

20) e.
A total institution is an organization in which a large number of like-situated individuals, cut off from the wider social world for an appreciable time together, lead an enclosed, formally administered way of life.

21) b.
Denial is the refusal to recognize external reality, and repression is the process by which thoughts that the conscious mind finds unacceptable are repressed from consciousness.

22) a.
Projection means that unacceptable qualities, feelings, thoughts or wishes are projected on to another person or thing.

23) b.
Displacement means that emotions, ideas or wishes are transferred from their original object to a more acceptable substitute.

24) a.
Magical undoing and isolation are other defence mechanisms associated with obsessive compulsive disorder.

25) b.
The attempt to undo has a magical quality and aims to reverse the reality of the original hostile thought or wish and recreate the past as if such intentions never existed.

26) c.
Regression is encouraged. The basic goals are structural reorganization of personality, resolution of unconscious conflicts, and insight into intrapsychic events. Symptom relief is an indirect result.

27) a.
Interpretation involves making something conscious that was previously unconscious.

28) e.
Condensation means that several unconscious impulses, wishes or feelings can be combined and attached to one manifest dream image; displacement means that energy associated with one object is diverted to a substitute object (projection was described as a special type of displacement); symbolic representation means that highly charged ideas will be represented by innocent images. Through secondary revision, primitive aspects of the dreams are organized to a more clear form.

29) d.
Dialectical therapy was developed by Linehan. Anthony Ryle developed cognitive analytic therapy.

30) e.
At the fourth session the therapist provides a summary of his/her understanding of the history and its meaning, and describes the maladaptive strategies (a diagram may be used). The patient feels understood and held and becomes less defensive. Sessions thereafter are usually unstructured, although homework is given.

31) e.
Transference is the displacement of attitudes and feelings originally experienced in relationships with people from the past onto the analyst.

32) c.
Yalom's curative factors include interpersonal learning, catharsis, group cohesiveness, insight, development of socializing techniques, existential awareness, universality, instillation of hope, altruism, corrective recapitulation of family group, guidance, and imitative behaviour.

33) c.
In a therapeutic community there are usually 20–30 members, who usually stay for 9–18 months. Main indications for therapeutic community are dissocial personality disorder and unstable personality disorder.

34) b.
Members learn about themselves through the reactions of other members, mutual help, directness and honesty. Group meetings are another principal feature.

35) c.
Excessive responsibility is associated with assumption of personal causality, e.g. 'I am responsible for all bad things'.

36) e.
The therapeutic relationship, listening, emotional release, information and advice, encouraging hope and persuasion are all important elements of supportive psychotherapy.

37) d.
The frequency and intensity of the problem situation, the patient's self-control, and the patient's environment are also assessed.

38) c.
Cognitive therapy for depression was developed by AT Beck.

39) b.
Neutralizing involves rehearsing a reassuring response to reduce anxiety.

40) e.
Social skills training is useful when skills may have been lost, possibly through disuse, in patients with chronic mental illness.

41) d.
Berne is associated with transactional analysis and Moreno with psychodrama.

42) a.
When marital problems result from conflict arising from a partner's sexual life, couple therapy is indicated.

43) e.
Sublimation is changing a socially objectionable aim to a socially acceptable one.

44) a.
Transference is shifting an emotional attitude from a past object or person to the therapist.

45) e.
The role of staff is to ensure a basic structure within which members of the community can interact.

46) e.
Obsessional symptoms occur when there is a regression to the anal stage of development

47) d.
Magical undoing is associated with obsessive compulsive disorder, and depression with turning against oneself and regression to the oral stage.

48) c.
Confrontation is not recommended; full physical examinations and investigations are necessary to rule out organic causes as well as to exclude serious medical problems. Positive reassurance and praising

healthy behaviour offer the patient a face-saving opportunity for rapid return to normal physical functioning.

49) b.
Cognitive behaviour therapy differs from dynamic psychotherapy in that it is not concerned with the way the disorder is developed.

50) b.
People develop safety behaviour as a way of reducing their immediate concerns but the long-term effect is to perpetuate the concerns.

Further reading

Gelder M, Harrison P, Cowen P. Chapter 22. In: *Shorter Oxford Textbook of Psychiatry*, 5th edn. Oxford: Oxford University Press, 2006.

Puri B, Hall A. Chapters 2 and 7. In: *Revision Notes in Psychiatry*, 2nd edn. London: Arnold/Hodder Education, 2004.

Sadock BJ, Sadock VA. Chapter 34. In: *Kaplan and Sadock's Comprehensive Textbook of Psychiatry*, 8th edn. Baltimore, MD: Lippincott Williams and Wilkins, 2005.

Smith EE, Bem DJ, Nolen-Hoeksema S. Chapters 14, 17 and 18. In: *Atkinson and Hilgard's Introduction to Psychology*, 14th edn. Florence, KY: Wadsworth Publishing Company, 2003.

5. Descriptive psychopathology: Questions

1) Empathy as a psychiatric term means:

   a. To feel the pain of the patient
   b. To be sympathetic to the patient's needs
   c. To describe the patient's symptoms objectively
   d. To understand the patient's subjective experience by 'putting oneself into the patient's shoes'
   e. Discussing the patient's problems in detail

2) Psychomotor agitation is characterized by:

   a. Verbally abusive behaviour
   b. Physically abusive behaviour
   c. Excessive activity with restlessness
   d. Restlessness and flight of ideas
   e. Restlessness and psychotic symptoms

3) Which of the following statements is true about 'stupor'?

   a. It is seen only in severe depression
   b. It can be caused by both psychiatric and neurological disorders
   c. Mutism is the diagnostic feature
   d. It never occurs in mania
   e. It never presents with excitement and over-activity

4) All of the following statements are true about REM sleep, except:

   a. It is associated with dreaming
   b. It is also known as paradoxical sleep
   c. An electroencephalogram (EEG) is characterized by sleep-spindles and K-complexes
   d. It is part of the normal sleep pattern
   e. An EEG shows relatively low-voltage activity

5) All of the following are true about somnambulism, except:

   a. It is more common in children
   b. It is more common in females
   c. It occurs in stages 3 and 4 of sleep
   d. It is not part of dreams
   e. It does not occur during REM

6) Which of the following is not true about narcolepsy?

a. It usually starts in childhood
b. It is often associated with cataplexy
c. It can be associated with hypnagogic hallucinations
d. It is usually not associated with organic brain pathology
e. It may be associated with sleep paralysis

7) Déjà vu:

a. Is characterized by a feeling of familiarity in unfamiliar circumstances
b. Is classified as a memory disorder
c. Is the opposite of jamais vu
d. Can be a presenting symptom of temporal lobe epilepsy
e. May be caused by cerebrovascular disease

8) All of the following statements are true about confabulation, except:

a. It is a falsification of memory occurring in clear consciousness
b. It is usually associated with organic brain damage
c. It is seen only in Korsakoff's syndrome
d. It has been described in patients with schizophrenia
e. Suggestibility is a common feature associated with it

9) All of the following are common features of Ganser syndrome, except:

a. Approximate answers
b. Psychopathic personality
c. Clouding of consciousness
d. Traumatic conversion features
e. Pseudohallucinations

10) All of the following are examples of sensory distortions, except:

a. Hyperacuss
b. Somatization
c. Micropsia
d. Macropsia
e. Dismegalopsia

11) Pareidolia:

a. Relates to hallucinatory phenomena
b. Is not uncommon in normal people
c. Can be provoked by psychoactive drugs
d. Is more common in children
e. Usually relates to visual phenomena

12) Which of the following statements is not true about hallucinations?

a. Are perceptions without objective stimuli
b. Occur in clear consciousness
c. Are perceived as true perceptions
d. Are common in schizophrenia
e. Are misinterpretations of external stimuli

13) All of the following statements are true about auditory hallucinations, except:

a. They are common in schizophrenia
b. They can occur in organic brain disorders
c. They always occur in the first person
d. They are not always distressing
e. They can occur in chronic alcohol abuse

14) Charles Bonnet syndrome is associated with all of the following, except:

a. More common in elderly people
b. Prominent visual hallucinations
c. Evidence of delirium
d. No evidence of psychosis
e. Reduced visual acuity

15) Delirium tremens is characterized by all of the following, except:

a. Alcoholic withdrawal
b. Lilliputian hallucinations
c. Affective illusions
d. Suggestibility
e. Auditory hallucinations giving a running commentary

16) Which of the following statements is true about pseudo-hallucinations?

a. They occur in objective space
b. They require voluntary creation
c. They have definite outlines
d. They are experienced as true perceptions
e. They are always suggestive of a morbid mental state

17) All of the following are examples of true hallucinations, except:

a. Pareidolia
b. Hypnagogic hallucinations
c. Extracampine hallucinations
d. Functional hallucinations
e. Reflex hallucinations

18) All of the following are examples of primary delusional phenomena, except:

   a. Autochthonous delusion
   b. Fregoli's delusion
   c. Delusional perception
   d. Delusional atmosphere
   e. Delusional memory

19) All of the following are true about delusions, except:

   a. They are false beliefs
   b. They are held with strong conviction
   c. They are out of keeping with the cultural background
   d. They feature a lack of insight
   e. They are diagnostic of schizophrenia

20) All of the following syndromes are examples of delusional misidentification, except:

   a. Capgras syndrome
   b. Fregoli's syndrome
   c. Intermetamorphosis syndrome
   d. Syndrome of subjective doubles
   e. De Clérambault's syndrome

21) Hypochondriac delusions:

   a. Can present as delusions of body odour
   b. Can present as delusions of infestation
   c. Can present as delusions of ugliness
   d. Are common in psychotic depression
   e. Never occur in schizophrenia

22) All of the following disorders are usually associated with overvalued ideas, except:

   a. Morbid jealousy
   b. Night terrors
   c. Dismorphophobia
   d. Anorexia nervosa
   e. Transsexualism

23) Which of the following is not an example of passivity phenomena?

   a. Formal thought disorder
   b. Thought insertion
   c. Thought withdrawal
   d. Thought broadcasting
   e. Made feelings

24) Which of the following disorders is unlikely to present as a stupor?

   a. Depression
   b. Obsessive compulsive disorder
   c. Mania
   d. Catatonic schizophrenia
   e. Epilepsy

25) Which of the following is not an example of compulsive rituals?

   a. Cleaning
   b. Counting
   c. Mannerisms
   d. Kleptomania
   e. Polydipsia

26) Which of the following is a compulsive ritual?

   a. Satyriasis
   b. Ambitendency
   c. Stereotypes
   d. Tics
   e. Posturing

27) Which of the following is not a feature of formal thought disorder as described by Schneider?

   a. Derailment
   b. Fusion
   c. Omission
   d. Substitution
   e. Mutism

28) Which of the following is not a negative symptom in schizophrenia?

   a. Delusions of control
   b. Blunting of affect
   c. Poverty of speech
   d. Loss of drive
   e. Social withdrawal

29) Which of the following is not a first-rank symptom of schizophrenia?

   a. Hallucinatory voices giving a running commentary
   b. Delusions of guilt
   c. Thought insertion
   d. Thought broadcast
   e. Somatic passivity

30) All of the following are examples of disorders of form of speech, except:

    a. Dysarthria
    b. Circumstantiality
    c. Flight of ideas
    d. Perseveration
    e. Thought blocking

31) Which of the following delusions is not common in depressive illness?

    a. Delusions of guilt
    b. Delusions of poverty
    c. Nihilistic delusions
    d. Hypochondriacal delusions
    e. Delusional misidentification

32) All of the following are true about obsessions, except:

    a. They are recurrent thoughts
    b. They are overvalued ideas
    c. They are difficult to resist
    d. They are recognized by the individual as absurd
    e. They may be associated with compulsions

33) Which of the following determine the form of a delusion?

    a. Type of illness
    b. Emotional state
    c. Social background
    d. Cultural background
    e. Religious beliefs

34) Which of the following is not characteristic of thought processes in schizophrenia?

    a. Derailment
    b. Fusion
    c. Drivelling
    d. Cirumstantiality
    e. Blocking

35) All of the following are language disorders caused by organic brain disease, except:

    a. Word deafness
    b. Word salad
    c. Word blindness
    d. Nominal dysphasia
    e. Jargon aphasia

36) All of the following statements are true about flight of ideas, except:

    a. It is common in mania
    b. It can be associated with pressure of speech
    c. It can present with muteness
    d. It is similar to retardation of thinking
    e. It is associated with distractibility

37) Which of the following is not true about verbigeration?

    a. It is repetition of words
    b. It is repetition of syllables
    c. It is similar to word salad
    d. It is seen in expressive dysphasia
    e. It causes communication difficulties

38) Which of the following is true about over-inclusive thinking?

    a. It is not associated with schizophrenia
    b. It is more common in patients with chronic schizophrenia
    c. It is not seen in the majority of schizophrenia patients
    d. It is similar to formal thought disorder
    e. There is a lack of connection between consecutive thoughts

39) Which of the following statements is not true about receptive dysphasia?

    a. It is an inability to understand spoken speech
    b. It is a loss of meaning of words
    c. It is difficulties with grammar
    d. It is impaired fluency of speech
    e. It is impaired writing and reading

40) Which of the following is not true about pure word dumbness?

    a. It is impaired understanding of spoken speech
    b. Writing ability is preserved
    c. Ability to understand writing is preserved
    d. Ability to respond to comments is preserved
    e. It is not local disturbance of speech muscles

41) Which of the following statements is not true about alexithymia?

    a. The term was coined by Sifneos
    b. It was originally introduced to describe psychosomatic disorders
    c. It is characterized by verbal expression of emotions
    d. It is associated with somatoform disorders
    e. It is associated with substance abuse disorders

42) Dissociative fugue states are characterized by all of the following, except:

    a. Sudden onset
    b. Wandering behaviour
    c. Change of identity
    d. Preserved everyday functioning
    e. Preserved memory

43) Clouding of consciousness is characterized by a disturbance in all of the following areas, except:

    a. Mood
    b. Attention
    c. Concentration
    d. Memory
    e. Orientation

44) Which of the following disorders is most likely to present with constructional apraxia?

    a. Lower motor neuron disease
    b. Spinal cord lesion at cervical level
    c. Pyramidal tract lesions
    d. Hypothalamic lesions
    e. Spinal cord lesions

45) Formal thought disorder in schizophrenia has been explained by all of the following terms, except:

    a. Acataphasia
    b. Logoclonia
    c. Loosening of associations
    d. Asyndesis
    e. Concrete thinking

46) Which of the following statements is true about autoscopy?

    a. It is also known as the double phenomena
    b. It is commonly seen in multiple personalities
    c. It means that the patient sees him/herself and knows that it is him/her
    d. It is diagnostic of schizophrenia
    e. It is seen in Charles Bonnet syndrome

47) Which of the following symptoms in schizophrenia is not a disturbance of boundaries of self?

    a. Third-person auditory hallucinations
    b. Hearing one's own thoughts out loud
    c. Delusions of control
    d. Delusions of persecution
    e. Thought broadcasting

48) Which of the following does not describe depersonalization?

    a. A subjective awareness of self
    b. Feelings of strangeness and unreality
    c. Loss of personal identity
    d. Feelings of thought emptiness
    e. Preserved insight

49) Which of the following is not seen in depersonalization?

    a. Emotional numbing
    b. Distortions in the experience of time
    c. Changes in the subjective experience of memory
    d. Loss of ego boundaries
    e. Heightened self-observation

50) Which of the following is not true about dysmorphophobia?

    a. It usually starts in middle age
    b. It is more common in females
    c. It is less common in married people or those living with partners
    d. There is frequent comorbidity with mood disorders
    e. There is a high rate of attempted suicide

51) Which of the following is not true about hypochondriasis?

    a. It is a well known disease
    b. Hypochondriacal symptoms are very common
    c. It can present with an undue concern about minor pain
    d. It can present with unreasonable fears about the likelihood of developing a serious illness
    e. Only a minority of patients are seen by psychiatrists

52) Which of the following does not characterize a dissociative disorder?

    a. Symptoms are psychogenic
    b. Selective amnesia is common
    c. Causation of the symptoms is always conscious
    d. Symptoms may carry some sort of advantage to the patient
    e. An environmental stress factor might be present

53) Which of the following is not a feature of anorexia nervosa?

    a. Body image distortion
    b. Self-induced weight loss
    c. Body weight 50% below the expected
    d. Amenorrhoea
    e. Delayed puberty

54) Which of the following is not true about phantom limb?

    a. It is a distortion of body image
    b. It is a rare occurrence in amputees
    c. The amputee is aware of the phantom limb in space
    d. The amputee can experience pain in the phantom limb
    e. The phantom limb can change size with the passage of time

55) In transsexualism, the preoccupation with changing one's sex is:

    a. An overvalued idea
    b. An obsession
    c. A phobia
    d. A delusion
    e. A delusional obsession

56) Which of the following is not true about phobias?

    a. A phobia is a fear of a particular object or situation
    b. The fear is out of proportion to the demands of the situation
    c. The subject understands that the fear is irrational and senseless
    d. The fear can be explained or reasoned away
    e. The fear leads to avoidance of the situation

57) Which of the following is a symptom of agoraphobia?

    a. Fear of leaving home
    b. Fear of speaking in public
    c. Fear of eating in the presence of others
    d. Fear of cats
    e. Fear of insects

58) Which of the following is not a motor disorder seen in schizophrenia?

    a. Catatonia
    b. Cataplexy
    c. Negativism
    d. Obstruction
    e. Automatic obedience

59) The term 'schizophrenia' was coined by:

    a. Kraepelin
    b. Schneider
    c. Bleuler
    d. Freud
    e. Jaspers

60) Which of the following is not a mood-congruent delusion in depression?

a. Delusion of guilt
b. Delusion of sin
c. Delusion of poverty
d. Delusion of control
e. Nihilist delusion

61) A patient with schizophrenia saying 'Everybody knows what I am thinking' is having:

a. Thought insertion
b. Thought broadcast
c. Thought withdrawal
d. Depersonalization
e. Somatic passivity

62) An elderly woman refusing to accept that her husband died of a heart attack 3 days ago is most likely to have:

a. Grief reaction
b. Morbid grief reaction
c. Depression
d. Psychosis
e. Delusional disorder

63) A patient with depression who says 'I feel as if I have no feelings' is having:

a. Somatic passivity
b. Thought withdrawal
c. Delusions of persecution
d. Depersonalization
e. Delusions of control

64) An elderly man suffering from depression who reports 'My heart has stopped and the blood is not flowing in my veins' is having which of the following phenomena?

a. Somatic passivity
b. Ideas of reference
c. Grandiose delusions
d. Persecutory delusions
e. Nihilism

65) Which of the following is not true about factitious disorder?

a. It features physical symptoms without an underlying cause
b. It features symptoms not under the voluntary control of the individual
c. It is a need to assume the sick role
d. It can present with pseudodementia
e. It has no obvious economic gain

66) A teenage girl seeking plastic surgery because of the small size of her breasts is likely to have which of the following?

a. Dysmorphophobia
b. Transsexualism
c. Anorexia nervosa
d. Hypomania
e. Phantom limb disorder

67) Delusions of infestation are also known as:

a. Münchausen syndrome
b. Folie imposée
c. Folie communiqué
d. Folie à deux
e. Ekbom syndrome

68) A patient who believes that strangers are actually close relatives in disguise is having which of the following?

a. Capgras syndrome
b. Syndrome of metamorphosis
c. Syndrome of subjective doubles
d. Fregoli's delusion
e. Persecutory delusions

69) Which of the following is not associated with pseudologia fantastica?

a. Untruthful statements
b. Grandiosity
c. Hypomania
d. Histrionic personality disorder
e. No evidence of organic illness

70) Doctor to a patient with Alzheimer's disease: 'How old are you?'
Patient: '67 years.'
Doctor: 'Where do you come from?'
Patient: '67 years.'
Which phenomenon is the patient exhibiting?

a. Obsessions
b. Compulsion
c. Rumination
d. Perseveration
e. Disorientation

71) A patient with schizophrenia reports that each time a fellow
patient sneezes he feels severe pain in his tummy. Which type of
hallucinatory phenomena is he exhibiting?

a. Extra-campine hallucinations
b. Reflex hallucinations
c. Functional hallucinations
d. Hypnagogic hallucinations
e. Pseudohallucinations

72) Which of the following does not fit into the description of Cotard's
syndrome?

a. Hypomania
b. Nihilistic delusions
c. Bizarre hypochondriacal delusions
d. Agitation
e. Lack of insight

73) Which of the following statements best describes the meaning of
anhedonia?

a. Somatic symptoms of pain
b. Inability to sleep
c. Loss of emotions
d. Apathy
e. Inability to experience pleasure

74) Which of the following is not true about autochthonous delusions?

a. They are primary delusions
b. They can be preceded by delusional mood
c. They can be a source of secondary delusions
d. They are also known as 'brain waves'
e. They are pathognomonic of schizophrenia

75) All of the following are recognized characteristics of schizoid personality disorder, except:

a. A greater likelihood of developing schizophrenia
b. Poor capacity to form social relationships
c. Emotional detachment
d. A tendency to break the law
e. Indifference to the feelings of other people

76) Unstable interpersonal relationships, impulsivity and recurrent suicidal behaviour are part of which of the following personality disorders?

a. Antisocial
b. Borderline
c. Schizoid
d. Paranoid
e. Histrionic

77) Which of the following is true about pseudohallucinations?

a. They cannot occur in normal people
b. They can be deliberately evoked
c. They arise in inner space
d. They are subject to conscious manipulation
e. They cannot have a definite outline and vivid detail

78) Which of the following is not a feature of catatonic schizophrenia?

a. Mitgehen
b. Logoclonia
c. Palilalia
d. Coprolalia
e. Stupor

79) Which of the following symptoms is unlikely to be seen in stupor?

a. Immobility
b. Muteness
c. Unresponsiveness
d. Unconsciousness
e. Open eyes

80) Ganser syndrome is commonly seen in:

a. Schizophrenia
b. Depression
c. Alzheimer's disease
d. Learning disabilities
e. Prisoners awaiting trial

81) Which of the following is not a feature of Tourette's syndrome?

a. Tics
b. Choreiform movements
c. Stereotype movements
d. Coprolalia
e. Head banging

82) Which of the following is not an illusion?

a. Micropsia
b. Macropsia
c. Pareidolia
d. Dysmegalopsia
e. Misinterpretation

5. Descriptive psychopathology: Answers

1) d.
Empathy involves proceeding through an organized series of questions, rephrasing and reiterating until one is sure of what the patient is describing.

2) c.
When psychomotor agitation is severe, the patient cannot sit for long but paces up and down.

3) b.
The key features of stupor include mutism, immobility and occasionally over-activity. Stupor can be caused by both psychiatric and neurological disorders.

4) c.
Sleep-spindles and K-complexes are normally seen in stage 2 of sleep. In REM sleep, a relatively low-voltage EEG is seen.

5) b.
Somnambulism is more common in males.

6) a.
Narcolepsy does not start in childhood but usually starts in adolescence.

7) d.
Déjà vu is not primarily a memory disorder.

8) c.
Although it is commonly seen in Korsakoff's syndrome, that is not the only condition in which confabulation is seen.

9) b.
Histrionic personality traits are more common in Ganser syndrome.

10) b.
Somatization is a process where physical symptoms are experienced in the absence of an adequate organic cause.

11) e.
Pareidolia involves illusions and not hallucinations.

12) e.
Hallucinations by definition occur without external stimuli.

13) c.
Auditory hallucinations can occur in a number of forms such as a running commentary, or voices talking to the patient in the first and third person.

14) c.
Delirium has to be excluded to diagnose Charles Bonnet syndrome.

15) e.
Auditory hallucinations giving a running commentary are not characteristic of delirium tremens but of schizophrenia.

16) b.
Pseudohallucinations require voluntary creation.

17) a.
Pareidolia involves illusions and not true hallucinations.

18) b.
Primary/autochthonous delusion is ultimately not understandable. Secondary delusions are understandable in terms of the patient's mood state and/or life history.

19) e.
Delusions are not diagnostic of schizophrenia and can be seen in other functional and organic disorders.

20) e.
De Clérambault's syndrome is also known as the delusion of love.

21) e.
Hypochondriacal delusions can occur in schizophrenia.

22) b.
An overvalued idea is an acceptable, comprehensible idea pursued by the patient beyond the boundaries of reason.

23) a.
Passivity experiences are those events in the realm of sensation, feeling, drive, and volition that are experienced as made or influenced by others. They have been well described as delusions of control.

24) b.
Stupor is a condition in which the patient is immobile, mute and unresponsive but appears to be fully conscious in that the eyes are usually open and follow external objects.

25) c.
Mannerisms are repeated involuntary movements that appear to be goal directed.

26) a.
Satyriasis is a compulsive need in the male to engage in sexual intercourse.

27) e.
Mutism is complete loss of speech.

28) a.
Delusions are classified as positive symptoms that respond well to treatment with neuroleptics compared with negative symptoms.

29) b.
Schneider described first-rank symptoms.

30) a.
Dysarthria is defined as a difficulty in the articulation of speech.

31) e.
Delusions in depression are usually mood-congruent.

32) b.
Obsessions are not overvalued ideas because the person retains insight.

33) a.
Unlike form, which is dictated by the type of illness, content is determined by the emotional, social and cultural background of the patient.

34) d.
Characteristically, circumstantial thinking occurs in epileptic patients, and is seen in other organic states and in mental retardation.

35) b.
Word salad occurs in schizophrenia.

36) d.
Retardation of thinking is the opposite of the flight of ideas and is commonly seen in depression.

37) c.

Word salad is characteristic of schizophrenia and verbigeration is seen in patients with expressive dysphasia.

38) c.

Fewer than half of patients with schizophrenia show over-inclusive thinking.

39) d.

Speech is fluent in receptive dysphasia.

40) a.

The ability to understand spoken speech is preserved in pure word dumbness.

41) c.

Alexithymia is characterized by difficulties in expressing and verbalizing emotions.

42) e.

Fugue states are characterized by amnesia.

43) a.

Clouding may be seen in many organic brain syndromes, drug and alcohol intoxication, head injury, and meningeal irritation.

44) e.

Spinal cord lesions are caused by cortical lesions.

45) b.

Logoclonia describes the spastic repetition of syllables that occurs in Parkinson's disease.

46) c.

Autoscopy is also known as phantom mirror image (seeing oneself and knowing that it is oneself).

47) d.

Delusion is a false unshakable belief.

48) c.

Depersonalization is not associated with loss or attenuation of personal identity.

49) d.

Loss of ego boundaries is seen in schizophrenia but the abnormality is not confined to schizophrenia.

50) a.
Dysmorphophobia usually starts in adolescence.

51) a.
Hypochondriasis is a symptom, not a disease.

52) c.
The causation of the symptoms is unconscious.

53) c.
The body weight is 15% lower than expected.

54) b.
Phantom limb phenomena occur in the majority of amputees.

55) a.
Transsexual people's belief that they are of the opposite sex is an overvalued idea taken to the extreme.

56) d.
In phobias the fear cannot be explained or reasoned away.

57) a.
A symptom of agoraphobia is a marked, consistent fear in or avoidance of at least two of the following situations: crowds, public places, travelling alone, travelling away from home.

58) b.
Cataplexy is seen in sleep disorder; in narcolepsy, the subject falls down because of sudden loss of muscle tone provoked by strong emotion.

59) c.
Swiss psychiatrist Eugen Bleuler coined the term 'schizophrenia' in 1911.

60) d.
Delusion of control is a passivity phenomenon seen in schizophrenia.

61) b.
Thought broadcast is also known as thought sharing or diffusion of thought.

62) a.
Morbid grief is associated with phobic avoidance, extreme guilt and anger, total lack of grieving, physical illness, and recurrent nightmares about the deceased.

63) d.
All the others are seen mainly in schizophrenia.

64) e.
Bizarre nihilistic and hypochondriachal delusions in elderly people are associated with Cotard's syndrome.

65) b.
Factitious disorder refers to self-inflicted signs and symptoms. It differs from malingering in that it does not bring any external reward such as financial compensation.

66) a.
Dysmorphophobia is sometimes described by schizophrenia patients.

67) e.
In Münchausen syndrome, the person intentionally fakes an illness. All the others are delusional disorders.

68) d.
False identification of strangers as familiar people occurs in Fregoli syndrome.

69) c.
Pseudologia fantastica is pathological lying.

70) d.
Perseveration is a sign of organic brain disease, perhaps the only pathognomonic sign in psychiatry.

71) b.
A hallucinatory form of synaesthesia, reflex hallucination is described as a stimulus in one sensory modality producing a hallucination in another.

72) a.
Cotard's syndrome is associated with agitated depression.

73) e.
Anhedonia is a core symptom of depression.

74) e.
Autochthonous delusions, although common in schizophrenia, are not pathognomonic of schizophrenia.

75) d.
Schizoid personalities do not have a tendency to break the law, which is a more common feature of antisocial personalities.

76) b.
Individuals with unstable personality disorder use less mature defence mechanisms, such as projection and denial.

77) c.
Pseudohallucinations arise in inner space as opposed to true hallucinations, which occur in objective space.

78) d.
Coprolalia is the obscene utterances commonly seen in Tourette's syndrome.

79) d.
The characteristic presentation of stupor is a lack of reaction to, and unawareness of surroundings. Unconsciousness is not a feature.

80) e.
In Ganser syndrome approximate answers, clouding of consciousness with disorientation, hysterical stigmata, recent history of head injury/typhus/severe emotional stress, pseudohallucinations and amnesia are present.

81) b.
Choreiform movements are not a feature of Tourette's syndrome but are commonly seen in Huntington's chorea and other neurological disorders.

82) e.
Misinterpretation means simply making a mistake.

Further reading

Fish FJ, Casey PR, Kelly B. *Fish's Clinical Psychopathology: Signs and Symptoms in Psychiatry*, 3rd edn. London: Royal College of Psychiatrists Publications, 2007.

Gelder M, Andreasen N, Lopez-Ibor J, Geddes J. Chapter 1. In: *New Oxford Textbook of Psychiatry*, 2nd edn. Oxford: Oxford University Press, 2009.

Oyebode F. *Sims' Symptoms in the Mind: An Introduction to Descriptive Psychopathology*, 4th edn. London: Saunders, 2008.

6. Psychopharmacology: antidepressants and anxiolytics: Questions

1) Tricyclic antidepressants:

   a. Are slowly absorbed from the gastrointestinal tract because they are not lipid soluble
   b. Have low protein binding
   c. Are subject to a low first-pass metabolism
   d. Have a plasma level linearly related to the clinical response
   e. Are metabolized in the liver and metabolites are predominantly excreted by the kidney

2) Tricyclic antidepressants:

   a. Commonly cause bradycardia and hypertension
   b. Frequently cause prolongation of PR and QT intervals on ECG
   c. Increase seizure threshold
   d. Increase the plasma concentration of carbamazepine
   e. When taken with monoamine oxidase inhibitors (MAOIs) increase MAOI-induced insomnia

3) Phenelzine has significant interaction with all of the following, except:

   a. Pethidine
   b. Methylphenidate
   c. Salbutamol
   d. Metformin
   e. ACE inhibitors

4) All of the following statements are true about serotonin syndrome, except:

   a. It may occur with a combination of tranylcypromine and L-tryptophan
   b. It is associated with myoclonus
   c. It can be associated with hypomania
   d. It can be fatal
   e. The treatment of choice is sodium dantrolene

5) All of the following statements are true, except:

a. First-pass metabolism could be avoided by sublingual administration of a drug
b. Highly protein-bound drugs are more likely to be secreted in the breast milk
c. Highly lipid-soluble drugs are more likely to be secreted in the breast milk
d. Highly water-soluble and ionized drugs cannot cross the blood–brain barrier easily
e. At steady state, the rate of removal of the drug equals the rate of input

6) Regarding pharmacokinetics:

a. A very high value of volume of distribution indicates that the drug is concentrated in the blood itself
b. The steady state of a drug is usually reached in 4–5 half-lives in first-order kinetics
c. Elimination of most drugs follows zero-order kinetics
d. Alcohol and phenytoin follow first-order kinetics
e. Tachyphylaxis is usually due to up-regulation or down-regulation of receptors

7) Which of the following statements is true about the action of drugs on receptors?

a. An agonist activates a receptor to produce an effect
b. An inverse agonist activates a receptor to produce an effect in the opposite direction to that of the well recognized agonist
c. An antagonist prevents the action of an agonist on a receptor or the subsequent response, but does not have any effect of its own
d. A partial agonist activates a receptor to produce a submaximal effect that antagonizes the action of a full agonist
e. All of the above

8) Foods not to be taken with tranylcypromine include all of the following, except:

a. Ricotta cheese
b. Red wine
c. Pickled herring
d. Broad bean pods
e. Fermented soya bean extract

9) Tranylcypromine is contraindicated in all of the following, except:

a. Severe hepatic impairment
b. Epilepsy
c. Hyperthyroidism
d. Phaeochromocytoma
e. Severe cerebrovascular disease

10) Moclobemide:

a. Is a reversible inhibitor of monoamine oxidase type A
b. Is licensed for use in social anxiety disorder
c. Causes less potentiation of pressor effects of tyramine than irreversible MAOIs
d. Should not be combined with SSRIs, because a serotonin syndrome may result
e. All of the above

11) Regarding special properties of drugs belonging to the tricyclic antidepressant class, all of the following are true, except:

a. Amoxapine produces significant blockade of dopamine D_2 receptors
b. Clomipramine is the most potent 5-HT reuptake inhibitor in the class
c. Lofepramine is a sedating antidepressant
d. Use of maprotiline in higher doses has been associated with a higher incidence of seizures
e. Desipramine causes insomnia

12) Recognized side-effects of tricyclic antidepressants (TCAs) include all of the following, except:

a. Worsening of glaucoma
b. Urinary incontinence
c. Heart block
d. Cognitive impairment
e. Sexual dysfunction

13) All of the following are true about selective serotonin reuptake inhibitors (SSRIs), except:

a. They are primarily eliminated by hepatic metabolism
b. Fluoxetine has the longest half-life in the class
c. They inhibit CYP450 enzymes, resulting in potential interactions with other drugs
d. Withdrawal reaction occurs more commonly with a longer half-life
e. The gastrointestinal side-effects are usually dose related

14) All of the following side-effects are usually associated with SSRIs, except:

a. Weight gain
b. Extra-pyramidal side-effects
c. Ejaculatory delay and anorgasmia
d. Hyponatraemia secondary to syndrome of inappropriate antidiuretic hormone (SIADH)
e. Increased risk of upper gastrointestinal bleeding

15) All of the following are true about SSRIs, except:

   a. They are recommended in combination therapy with MAOIs in resistant depression
   b. They may cause myoclonus and seizures when used with lithium and tryptophan
   c. They may potentiate the induction of extra-pyramidal movement disorders by antipsychotic drugs
   d. Serotonin toxicity may occur if combined with sumatryptan
   e. They may increase the plasma levels of risperidone

16) All of the following are true statements, except:

   a. Priapism is a serious side-effect of trazodone
   b. Nefazodone elevates the plasma levels of haloperidol
   c. Reboxetine is a reversible inhibitor of MAO-A
   d. Mainserin can cause fatal agranulocytosis
   e. L-tryptophan is associated with eosinophilia–myalgia syndrome

17) Venlafaxine:

   a. Is a noradrenaline and serotonin specific antidepressant (NASSA)
   b. Is recommended for combined use with moclobemide in resistant depression
   c. May cause postural hypotension and dose-related hypertension
   d. Is more toxic in overdose than tricyclic antidepressants
   e. May cause high plasma sodium levels

18) L-tryptophan:

   a. Has direct action on 5-HT receptors
   b. Has a low protein binding
   c. Can enhance the antidepressant effects of MAOIs
   d. Is non-sedative
   e. High doses are associated with decrease in slow-wave sleep

19) All of the following properties of SSRIs are thought to be mediated mainly by the subtypes of 5-HT receptors, except:

   a. $5-HT_1$ receptor: antidepressant action
   b. $5-HT_2$ receptor: anxiolytic action
   c. $5-HT_2$ receptor: sexual dysfunction
   d. $5-HT_3$ receptor: nausea
   e. $5-HT_3$ receptor: headache

20) St John's wort:

   a. Increases the anticoagulant effect of warfarin
   b. Reduces the plasma concentration of amitriptyline
   c. Reduces the serotoninergic effects of SSRIs
   d. Increases plasma concentration of aripiprazole
   e. Increases plasma concentration of digoxin

21) All of the following are true about lithium, except:

   a. It is the smallest alkaline cation
   b. It acts through second messengers
   c. It is not metabolized in the body
   d. It is highly protein bound
   e. It is reabsorbed in the proximal tubule

22) In relation to lithium:

   a. Lithium is transported in the proximal tubule in competition with sodium
   b. When the proximal tubule absorbs more water, lithium absorption decreases
   c. Dehydration causes plasma lithium concentration to fall
   d. Hyponatraemia causes plasma lithium concentration to fall
   e. Thiazide diuretics cause plasma lithium concentration to fall

23) All of the following are adverse renal effects of lithium, except:

   a. Nephrogenic diabetes insipidus
   b. Minimal change glomerulonephritis
   c. Renal cell carcinoma
   d. Reduced glomerular filtration rate (GFR) and renal failure
   e. Interstitial nephritis

24) Excretion of lithium is reduced by all of the following, except:

   a. ACE inhibitors
   b. Indomethacin
   c. Acetazolamide
   d. Furosemide
   e. Amiloride

25) All of the following statements are true about lithium, except:

    a. There is an increased risk of hypothyroidism when lithium is given with amiodarone

    b. Carbamazepine increases plasma concentration of lithium and causes neurotoxicity

    c. There is an increased risk of extra-pyramidal side-effects and neuro-toxicity when lithium is given with antipsychotics

    d. There is an increased risk of extra-pyramidal side-effects when lithium is given with metoclopramide

    e. Antacids and theophylline cause increased excretion of lithium

26) All of the following are recognized side-effects of lithium, except:

    a. Weight loss

    b. Hair loss

    c. Hypothyroidism

    d. Hyperparathyroidism

    e. Osteoporosis

27) The effects of lithium on thyroid include:

    a. Interference with iodine uptake

    b. Interference with tyrosine iodination

    c. Interference with release of T3 and T4

    d. Increased levels of thyroid-stimulating hormone (TSH)

    e. All of the above

28) All of the following statements are true, except:

    a. Lithium treatment may cause remission of pre-existing psoriasis

    b. The thyroid dysfunction as a result of lithium treatment occurs more commonly in women

    c. Weight gain as a result of lithium treatment occurs more commonly in women

    d. Osteoporosis as a result of lithium treatment occurs more commonly in women

    e. Propanol may reduce tremor associated with lithium treatment

29) Regarding treatment with lithium in pregnancy:

    a. The absolute risk of the cardiac malformation Ebstein's anomaly is very high

    b. The period of maximum risk is second trimester

    c. Neonatal goitre can occur

    d. At parturition, diuresis may lead to reduced serum levels of lithium

    e. Lithium is safe in breastfeeding

30) In lithium toxicity all of the following are true, except:

    a. Early clinical signs may include apathy
    b. Constipation is a usual sign
    c. Convulsions and coma occur
    d. Concentrations above 2 mmol/litre are usually associated with serious toxicity
    e. Haemodialysis may be needed

31) The pharmacodynamic properties of carbamazepine include:

    a. Binding to voltage-dependent sodium channels and prolonging their inactivation
    b. Reducing voltage-dependent calcium channel activation and therefore synaptic transmission
    c. Reduction of current through NMDA receptor channels
    d. Competitive antagonism of adenosine A_1 receptors
    e. All of the above

32) Significant pharmacodynamic interaction occurs between carbamazepine and:

    a. Antipsychotics
    b. TCAs
    c. Calcium channel blockers
    d. Lithium
    e. All of the above

33) Carbamazepine:

    a. Commonly causes agranulocytosis
    b. Is safe in disturbances in cardiac conduction
    c. Usually causes clinical hypothyroidism
    d. Is associated with high sodium states
    e. Induces its own metabolism

34) In bipolar illness, which of the following is a predictor of good response to treatment with lithium?

    a. Family history of bipolar illness
    b. Prominent depressive features
    c. Psychotic symptoms
    d. Rapid cycling
    e. None of the above

35) Valproate:

    a. Induces hepatic microsomal enzymes
    b. Has many active metabolites
    c. Is not useful in longer-term prophylaxis of bipolar disorder
    d. Is a drug of choice in generalized absences and myoclonic epilepsy
    e. Has low protein binding

36) Valproate:

    a. Is known to decrease synaptic levels of GABA
    b. Is a preferred choice over lithium in pregnancy
    c. Is not useful in patients with bipolar illness who are unresponsive to lithium and carbamazepine
    d. Is not secreted in breast milk
    e. Is not safe in hepatic dysfunction

37) Common side-effects of valproate include:

    a. Sedation
    b. Fatal hepatic toxicity
    c. Thrombocytopenia
    d. Acute pancreatitis
    e. Amenorrhoea

38) Valproate increases the concentration of all of the following, except:

    a. Erythromycin
    b. Lamotrigine
    c. Phenytoin
    d. Diazepam
    e. Barbiturates

39) All of the following are true about lamotrigine, except:

    a. It blocks voltage-dependent calcium channels
    b. It reduces the release of excitatory neurotransmitter glutamate
    c. It is effective as a monotherapy in the treatment of bipolar depression
    d. Adverse effects include Stevens–Johnson syndrome
    e. Plasma levels can be lowered by carbamazepine

40) All of the following are true about gabapentin, except:

    a. It is a GABA receptor agonist
    b. It increases GABA turnover in the brain
    c. It has a sedating profile
    d. It has anxiolytic properties
    e. It is excreted entirely by the kidney

41) Psychostimulants:

   a. Include methylphenidate and cocaine
   b. Increase the release and block the reuptake of dopamine and noradrenaline
   c. Are used to treat narcolepsy
   d. Are useful in the hyperkinetic syndrome of childhood
   e. All of the above

42) Benzodiazepines:

   a. Increase the affinity of $GABA_A$ receptor for GABA
   b. Are strongly bound to the plasma proteins
   c. Are lipophilic
   d. Agonist effects can be reversed by flumazenil
   e. All of the above

43) Buspirone:

   a. Is a partial agonist at 5-HT_{1A} receptors
   b. Is an agonist at dopamine D_2 receptors
   c. Is useful in treating benzodiazepine withdrawal
   d. Tolerance and dependence occur commonly
   e. Is highly sedative

44) Which of the following statements is true about hypnotics?

   a. Zopiclone produces more changes in sleep architecture than benzodiazepines
   b. Zolpidem acts at benzodiazepine receptors
   c. Zaleplon does not cause a dependence syndrome
   d. Taste disturbance is a rare side-effect of zopiclone
   e. Clomethiazole is safe to use in alcohol-dependent patients who continue to drink

45) Flumazenil:

   a. Is a benzodiazepine antagonist, producing few pharmacological effects by itself
   b. Is available only for intravenous use
   c. Is useful in reversing acute toxicity produced by benzodiazepines
   d. Carries a risk of provoking acute benzodiazepine withdrawal
   e. All of the above

46) Regarding benzodiazepines:

a. Actions are mediated through specific receptor sites on GABA receptors
b. Benzodiazepines with high potency and shorter half-lives are more associated with dependence and withdrawal
c. Benzodiazepines can cause respiratory depression when combined with clozapine
d. Withdrawal syndrome is associated epileptic seizures
e. All of the above

47) All of the following statements are true about treatment with benzodiazepines, except:

a. Dependence is likely in patients with a history of alcohol or drug abuse
b. Dependence is likely in patients with marked personality disorders
c. Lorazepam and oxazepam may be preferred in patients with hepatic impairment
d. They are safe in myasthenia gravis
e. They may cause paradoxical increase in aggression

48) Safe psychotropic medications in porphyria include:

a. Amphetamine
b. TCAs
c. MAOIs
d. Mianserin
e. Barbiturates

49) All of the following are true about anxiolytics, except:

a. Propranolol is effectively used to treat bodily symptoms of anxiety
b. Meprobamate is less hazardous in overdose than benzodiazepines
c. Barbiturate withdrawal may be fatal
d. Benzodiazepines cause amnesia
e. Buspirone has no affinity for benzodiazepine receptors

50) Drugs useful in narcolepsy include all of the following, except:

a. Dexamphetamine
b. Methylphenidate
c. Modafinil
d. Sibutramine
e. Tricyclic antidepressants

6. Psychopharmacology: antidepressants and anxiolytics: Answers

1) e.
Tricyclic antidepressants have rapid absorption, are highly lipophilic and have high protein binding.

2) b.
Tricyclic antidepressants commonly cause tachycardia and hypotension, and decrease seizure threshold and the plasma concentration of carbamazepine. When taken with MAOIs, they decrease MAOI-induced insomnia, and increase postural hypotension and weight gain.

3) c.
Pethidine is used for CNS excitation or depression and may cause impaired consciousness and coma; methylphenidate is used for hypertensive crisis; metformin is used for hypoglycaemia; ACE inhibitors are used for enhanced hypotensive effect.

4) e.
Sodium dantrolene is used in patients with neuroleptic malignant syndrome (NMS) and malignant hyperthermia. In 5-HT syndrome, treatment is mainly supportive and all medications should be stopped.

5) b.
Protein binding can influence the drug's biological half-life in the body.

6) b.
A low volume of distribution indicates that the drug is concentrated in the blood itself; elimination of most drugs follows first-order kinetics, but alcohol and phenytoin follow zero-order kinetics. Tachyphylaxis is the very rapid development of tolerence, most often due to desensitization of the drug receptors (e.g. benzodiazepines). Tolerance can also develop from slower adaptive changes like up-regulation of receptors with antagonists and down-regulation with agonists.

7) e.
An agonist is a compound that mimics the action of a neurotransmitter; an antagonist is a compound that blocks or inhibits the action of a neurotransmitter.

8) a.
All cheeses except cream, cottage and ricotta should be avoided.

9) b.
Tranylcypromine is an MAOI with an amphetamine-like stimulating effect that may be helpful in patients with anergia and retardation.

10) e.
Moclobemide is the most recently developed MAOI.

11) c.
TCAs inhibit the reuptake of both 5-HT and noradrenaline.

12) b.
TCAs cause retention of urine.

13) d.
Paroxetine has the shortest half-life.

14) a.
SSRIs inhibit the reuptake of 5-HT with high potency and selectivity.

15) a.
Simultaneous administration of SSRIs and MAOIs causes 5-HT toxicity syndrome (the serotonin syndrome) with agitation, hyperpyrexia, rigidity, myoclonus, coma and death. Other drugs (lithium, tryptophan, 5-HT receptor agonist sumatryptan) that increase brain 5-HT function also cause similar reactions.

16) c.
Reboxetine is a selective noradrenaline reuptake inhibitor.

17) c.
Venlafaxine is a selective serotonin and noradrenaline reuptake inhibitor (SNRI). Combination with moclobemide causes serotonin syndrome. Preliminary evidence suggests that it is less toxic in overdose than tricyclic antidepressants.

18) c.
L-tryptophan is a precursor of 5-HT. It is highly protein binding. It can cause serotonin syndrome with SSRIs and MAOIs. It is a sedative. High doses are associated with an increase in slow-wave sleep.

19) b.
$5\text{-}HT_1$ receptor, anxiolytic; $5\text{-}HT_2$ receptor, insomnia, agitation and sexual dysfunction.

20) b.
St John's wort reduces the anticoagulant effect of warfarin, increases the serotoninergic effects of SSRIs, reduces the plasma concentration of

aripiprazole, digoxin, simvastatin, theophylline, carbamazepine and phenytoin, and reduces the contraceptive effects of oestrogen and progesterone.

21) d.
Lithium is not bound to proteins.

22) a.
When the proximal tubule absorbs more water, lithium absorption decreases; dehydration, hyponatraemia and thiazide diuretics cause plasma lithium concentration to fall.

23) c.
Lithium blocks the effects of ADH on the renal tubule.

24) c.
Insufficient intake of water in patients with lithium-induced polyuria may lead to a rapid lowering of lithium clearance and, hence, to a rise in the serum lithium concentration and development of intoxication.

25) b.
Carbamazepine when given with lithium causes neurotoxicity without increasing the plasma concentration of lithium.

26) a.
Weight gain is a side-effect of lithium.

27) e.
Thyroid enlargement occurs in 5% and hypothyroidism in 20% of women treated with lithium.

28) a.
Lithium treatment may cause exacerbation of pre-existing psoriasis.

29) c.
The absolute risk of Ebstein's anomaly (right ventricular hypoplasia and tricuspid valve insufficiency) is low at 1:1000, but the relative risk is 10–20 times higher than control. The period of maximum risk is the first trimester (2–6 weeks). Neonatal goitre, hypotonia and arrhythmias can occur. Parturition diuresis may lead to increased serum levels of lithium, leading to toxicity because of the reduced plasma volume and redistribution.

30) b.
Diarrhoea, vomiting, tremor, etc. are the usual signs of lithium toxicity.

31) e.
Carbamazepine is effective as an antiepileptic, as prophylaxis of bipolar disorder, and in management of acute mania.

32) e.
Carbamazepine is a strong inducer of hepatic microsomal enzymes.

33) e.
Agranulocytosis is a serious but rare side-effect; carbamazepine is contraindicated in cardiac conduction abnormalities, lowers plasma thyroxine concentration (though clinical hypothyroidism is unusual) and is associated with low sodium states.

34) a.
b, c and d are indicators of poor response.

35) d.
Unlike carbamazapine, valproate does not induce hepatic microsomal enzymes and, if anything, tends to delay the metabolism of other drugs.

36) e.
Valproate is 80–95% protein bound; it has no active metabolites; it does not induce hepatic enzymes but delays metabolism of some drugs that are metabolized in the liver; it is hepatotoxic; it increases synaptic levels of GABA and causes major congenital malformations (e.g. spina bifida, neural tube defects in up to 5%); folate reduces the risk. Up to 10% of serum concentration is secreted in breast milk.

37) a.
The others are less common side-effects.

38) a.
Valproate reduces the concentration of erythromycin.

39) a.
Lamotrigine blocks voltage-dependent sodium channels.

40) a.
Gabapentin was developed as a structural analogue of GABA but it has no activity on GABA receptors or the GABA transporter.

41) e.
Psychostimulants include caffeine, amphetamine, methylphenidate, cocaine, etc.

42) e.
Benzodiazepines pass readily into the brain.

43) a.
Buspirone is an antagonist at D_2; tolerance and dependence will not occur usually; it is not a sedative but may cause light-headedness.

44) b.
Zopiclone produces fewer changes in sleep architecture. Taste disturbance is common.

45) e.
Flumazenil does not antagonize the central nervous system effects of drugs affecting GABA-ergic neurons other than the benzodiazepine receptor (including ethanol, barbiturates and general anaesthetics) and does not reverse the effects of opioids.

46) e.
Benzodiazepines are anxiolytic, sedative and hypnotic, muscle relaxant, and anticonvulsant.

47) d.
Benzodiazepines are contraindicated in myasthenia gravis (increased respiratory depression).

48) d.
Drugs that lead to increased activity of the hepatic P450 system, such as phenobarbital, sulfonamides, oestrogens and alcohol, are associated with porphyria.

49) b.
Meprobamate is less effective and more hazardous in overdose than benzodiazepines and can induce dependence.

50) d.
Sibutramine is a centrally acting appetite suppressant used in treatment for obesity. TCAs and SSRIs do not affect the sleep disorder but may reduce the frequency of cataplexy.

Further reading

British National Formulary. *BNF 57*. London: Pharmaceutical Press. Also available at: www.bnf.org/bnf.
Cookson J, Taylor D, Katona C. *Use of Drugs in Psychiatry*, 5th edn. London: Gaskell, 2002.

Gelder M, Andreasen N, Lopez-Ibor J, Geddes J. Chapter 21. In: *New Oxford Textbook of Psychiatry*, 2nd edn. Oxford: Oxford University Press, 2009.

Rosenbaum JF, Arana GW, Hyman SE, Labbate LA, Fava M. *Handbook of Psychiatric Drug Therapy*, 5th edn. Baltimore, MD: Lippincott Williams and Wilkins, 2005.

Sadock BJ, Sadock VA. Chapter 36. In: *Kaplan and Sadock's Synopsis of Psychiatry*, 10th edn. Baltimore, MD: Lippincott Williams and Wilkins, 2008.

Stahl SM. *Stahl's Essential Psychopharmacology: Neuroscientific Basis and Practical Applications*, 3rd edn. Cambridge: Cambridge University Press, 2008.

7. Psychopharmacology: antipsychotics and organic disorders: Questions

1) All of the following are true about pharmacodynamics of antipsychotics, except:

   a. The antipsychotic effect is most closely correlated with the drug's affinity with D_2 receptors
   b. The antipsychotic effects may derive from inhibition of dopaminergic neurotransmission in the mesolimbic–cortical tract
   c. The Parkinsonian side-effects derive from inhibition of dopaminergic neurotransmission in the nigrostriatal tract
   d. The endocrine side-effects derive from inhibition of dopaminergic neurotransmission in the tuberoinfudibular tract
   e. The antipsychotic effect of clozapine is correlated with its tendency to occupy 80–100% of D_2 receptors

2) The following antipsychotics are correctly matched with their chemical class, except:

   a. Chlorpromazine–Aliphatic phenothiazine
   b. Thioridazine–Piperidine phenothizine
   c. Trifluperazine–Piperazine phenothiazine
   d. Haloperidol–Diphenylbutylpiperidines
   e. Flupenthixol–Thioxanthines

3) All of the following are true about chlorpromazine, except:

   a. Blockade of α_1-adrenoreceptors gives it a sedating profile
   b. Blockade of histamine H_1-receptors gives it a sedating profile
   c. Blockade of α_1-adrenoreceptors causes hypertension
   d. Muscarinic cholinergic receptor blockade produces urinary retention and constipation
   e. Muscarinic cholinergic receptor blockade protects against Parkinsonian symptoms

4) Which of the following statements is true about antipsychotics?

   a. Thioridazine is a potent muscarinic antagonist with low incidence of movement disorders
   b. Acute dystonic reaction occurs more commonly with chlorpromazine than with haloperidol
   c. Histamine H_2 blockade causes hyperprolactinaemia
   d. Haloperidol is highly sedative
   e. Pimozide is safe in cardiac arrhythmias

5) All of the following are true about substituted benzamides, except:

    a. They include amisulpride
    b. They are highly selective D_2 receptor antagonists
    c. They cause hyperprolactinaemia
    d. They are more likely to cause sedation
    e. They lack anticholinergic properties

6) Risperidone has high affinity to all receptors, except:

    a. D_2 dopamine receptors
    b. $5\text{-}HT_{2A}$ receptors
    c. α_1-adrenergic receptors
    d. α_2-adrenergic receptors
    e. Muscarinic cholinergic receptors

7) All of the following are well known side-effects of risperidone, except:

    a. Postural hypotension
    b. Diarrhoea
    c. Galactorrhoea
    d. Sexual dysfunction
    e. Weight gain

8) Atypical antipsychotics:

    a. Are associated with an increased risk of stroke in elderly patients with dementia
    b. May cause tardive dyskinesia on long-term administration
    c. Can cause hyperglycaemia and sometimes diabetes
    d. Rarely cause neuroleptic malignant syndrome
    e. All of the above

9) Significant interaction occurs between aripiprazole and all the following medications, except:

    a. Fluoxetine
    b. Carbamazepine
    c. Ketoconazole
    d. Antivirals
    e. Lithium

10) With which of the following are anticholinergic side-effects more common?

    a. Clozapine
    b. Amisulpride
    c. Risperidone
    d. Olanzapine
    e. Quetiapine

11) With which of the following does most marked α_1 blockade occur?

a. Clozapine
b. Amisulpride
c. Risperidone
d. Olanzapine
e. Quetiapine

12) Hyperprolactinaemia commonly occurs in treatment with all antipsychotics, except:

a. Chlorpromazine
b. Clozapine
c. Sulpiride
d. Haloperidol
e. Risperidone

13) All of the following are common side-effects of clozapine, except:

a. Constipation
b. Hypersalivation
c. Dry mouth
d. Priapism
e. Sedation

14) All of the following are true about treatment with clozapine, except:

a. It is almost free of extra-pyramidal symptoms (EPS)
b. It may improve existing tardive dyskinesia (TD)
c. It causes 95% of agranulocytosis within the first 6 months of treatment
d. Occurrence of agranulocytosis is approximately 5%
e. It is indicated in psychosis in Parkinson's disease

15) Olanzapine:

a. Is a dibenzothiazepine
b. Is a stronger receptor antagonist than risperidone
c. Blocks the histamine H_1 receptor
d. Commonly causes abnormalities of the QT interval
e. All of the above

16) Acute dystonic reaction:

a. Occurs later on in long-term treatment with antipsychotics
b. Is more common in elderly people
c. Is more likely to occur with chlorpromazine than haloperidol
d. Can be easily mistaken for histrionic behaviour
e. Is exacerbated by anticholinergic agents

17) All of the following are true about akathisia, except:

    a. It usually occurs in the first 2 weeks of antipsychotic treatment
    b. It is reliably controlled by anti-Parkinsonian drugs
    c. Treatment with beta-blockers can be helpful
    d. Treatment with benzodiazepines can be helpful
    e. Reduction in the dose of antipsychotic can be helpful

18) Among atypical antipsychotics:

    a. Olanzapine is safe in angle closure glaucoma
    b. Clozapine causes hyperprolactinaemia
    c. Amisulpride is excreted unchanged by the kidney
    d. QT prolongation is a common side-effect of aripiprazole
    e. Sertindole is safe to use in cardiac conduction abnormalities

19) Among the following antipsychotics, secretion in the breast is lowest with:

    a. Sulpiride
    b. Clozapine
    c. Olanzapine
    d. Quetiapine
    e. Risperidone

20) Which of the following statements is true?

    a. Clozapine is safe to give in pregnancy
    b. Galactorrhoea is more common with risperidone than olanzapine
    c. Zotepine is safe in cardiac arrythmias
    d. Anticholinergic drugs should be given regularly to people receiving antipsychotics to reduce side-effects
    e. Clozapine is contraindicated in Parkinsonism

21) Parkinsonian side-effects of neuroleptics:

    a. Occur as a consequence of mesocortical dopamine D_2 receptor occupancy
    b. Always appear a few months after the drug has been taken
    c. Do not respond to anti-Parkinsonian treatments
    d. May be treated with trihexyphenidyl
    e. Occur in 90% of patients treated with dopamine receptor antagonists

22) Parkinsonian side-effects of neuroleptics

    a. Are more common in women
    b. Are more common after the age of 40
    c. Include rabbit syndrome
    d. May continue after stopping the neuroleptics
    e. All of the above

23) Antipsychotics:

  a. Are mainly absorbed from the jejunum
  b. Are highly protein bound
  c. Can be used for treating behavioural symptoms of dementia
  d. May cause hypothermia in the elderly
  e. All of the above

24) Groups at higher risk of tardive dyskinesia include all of the following, except:

  a. Women
  b. Elderly people
  c. People with diffuse brain damage
  d. People with mood disorder
  e. People with personality disorder

25) Which of the following is true of tardive dyskinesia?

  a. Patients always recover when the neuroleptic is stopped
  b. It is more common in long-term treatment
  c. It occurs in 50% of patients treated with typical neuroleptics
  d. It will not occur in patients treated with atypical antipsychotics
  e. It improves when treated with anticholinergic anti-Parkinsonian drugs

26) Which of the following is true of tardive dyskinesia?

  a. It is characterized by chewing and sucking movements
  b. The limbs and the muscles of respiration may also be involved
  c. It may be seen in patients taking metoclopramide
  d. It is aggravated frequently by stopping the antipsychotic drug
  e. All of the above

27) The clinical picture of neuroleptic malignant syndrome includes all of the following, except:

  a. Gradual onset of generalized muscular hypertonicity
  b. Stupor
  c. Hyperpyrexia with fluctuating autonomic dysfunction
  d. Increased creatinine phosphokinase levels
  e. Decreased white cell count

28) Which of the following is true of neuroleptic malignant syndrome?

  a. It can be lethal in up to 50% of patients
  b. Risk is decreased in combined lithium and antipsychotic treatment
  c. It will not occur with clozapine
  d. It may cause myoglobinuria, leading to renal failure
  e. Patients who survive usually have residual disability

29) Medications used to treat neuroleptic malignant syndrome include:

    a. Dantrolene
    b. Diazepam
    c. Bromocriptine
    d. Amantadine
    e. All of the above

30) Fluoxetine increases the plasma concentration of all of the following, except:

    a. Clozapine
    b. Haloperidol
    c. Risperidone
    d. Olanzapine
    e. Zotepine

31) Carbamazepine accelerates the metabolism of:

    a. Clozapine
    b. Haloperidol
    c. Quetiapine
    d. Olanzapine
    e. All of the above

32) Anticholinergic anti-Parkinsonian drugs may cause all of the following, except:

    a. Exacerbation of glaucoma
    b. Exacerbation of tardive dyskinesia
    c. Dry mouth
    d. Diarrhoea
    e. Dependence

33) Impaired glucose tolerance is associated with:

    a. Phenothiazines
    b. Clozapine
    c. Olanzapine
    d. Risperidone
    e. All of the above

34) Sexual dysfunction is a side-effect of:

    a. Phenothiazines
    b. Haloperidol
    c. Risperidone
    d. Amisulpride
    e. All of the above

35) All of the following statements are true, except:

   a. Amisulpride causes SIADH
   b. SSRIs are associated with an increased risk of gastrointestinal bleed
   c. TCAs cause hyperglycaemia
   d. Atomoxetine is safe to use in hepatic impairment
   e. Modafenil is used to treat obstructive sleep apnoea syndrome

36) It is reported that in clinical practice the most effective drug for Tourette's syndrome is:

   a. Haloperidol
   b. Domperidone
   c. Atomoxetine
   d. Amantadine
   e. Rivastigmine

37) Regarding drugs used to treat substance misuse problems, all of the following are true, except:

   a. Acamprosate is safe to use in hepatic impairment
   b. Disulfiram is safe to recommend in controlled drinking
   c. Taste disturbance is a rare side-effect of bupropion
   d. In opioid dependence, buprenorphine may precipitate withdrawal reactions due to its partial antagonist properties
   e. Lofexidine is not useful in alleviating symptoms of opioid withdrawal

38) Features of opioid withdrawal include all of the following, except:

   a. Sweating
   b. Running eyes and nose
   c. Yawning
   d. Fast pulse and raised blood pressure
   e. Constricted pupils

39) All of the following are true statements about drugs used in opiate misuse, except:

   a. Methadone is a synthetic opiate with a high dependency potential and low lethal dose
   b. Buprenorphine undergoes extensive first-pass metabolism
   c. Lofexidine is a peripherally acting α_2-adrenergic antagonist
   d. Naltrexone causes increased sweating and lacrimation
   e. Naloxone is used to reverse neonatal respiratory depression resulting from opioid administration to the mother during labour

40) All of the following are true about pharmacokinetics in ageing, except:

    a. Gastric pH increases
    b. Intestinal perfusion decreases
    c. Total body water and lean body mass increase
    d. Total body fat increases more markedly in women than men
    e. The free or unbound percentage of albumin-bound drugs increases

41) Regarding drugs for dementia:

    a. Acetylcholinesterase-inhibiting drugs are not useful in dementia associated with Parkinson's disease
    b. Donepezil is an irreversible acetylcholinesterase inhibitor
    c. Galantamine is a reversible inhibitor of acetylcholinesterase with nicotinic receptor agonist properties
    d. Rivastigmine is a competitive inhibitor of acetylcholinesterase
    e. Memantine is an NMDA receptor agonist

42) Which of the following anti-dementia medications is safe to use in supraventricular cardiac conduction abnormalities?

    a. Tacrine
    b. Donepezil
    c. Rivastigmine
    d. Galantamine
    e. Memantine

43) All of the following are antimuscarinic drugs used in Parkinsonism, except:

    a. Amantadine
    b. Benzatropine
    c. Orphenadrine
    d. Procyclidine
    e. Trihexyphenidyl

44) Common side-effects of levodopa include all of the following, except:

    a. Psychosis
    b. Hypersexuality
    c. Confusion
    d. Insomnia
    e. Depression

45) Psychosis is a known side-effect of all of the following, except:

    a. Metronidazole
    b. Tramadol
    c. Prednisolone
    d. Prochlorperazine
    e. Bromocriptine

46) You are asked to assess a 17-year-old boy brought to the A&E Department by his friends after a party. He is extremely agitated and tells you that 'aliens' are after him and they had put some 'radioactive things' in his body, which he could sense as 'crawling' underneath his skin. On examination he has dilated pupils and tachycardia. The most probable diagnosis is:

    a. Morphine withdrawal
    b. Cocaine intoxication
    c. Amphetamine intoxication
    d. Use of 'magic mushrooms'
    e. Cannabis abuse

47) You are asked to assess a 54-year-old man brought to the A&E Department by paramedics. You found him waiting in front of the A&E help desk believing that it was the local pub. It was reported that he had been wandering near a caravan park early in the morning. On examination he was found to be disorientated in time, and had an ataxic gait. He also had nystagmus and external rectus palsy. The treatment of choice is:

    a. Intravenous glucose
    b. Intramuscular haloperidol
    c. Chlordiazepoxide reducing regime
    d. Intravenous thiamine
    e. Intravenous naloxone

48) All of the following are true about pharmacological effects on the neurophysiology of the brain, except:

    a. Benzodiazepines decrease REM sleep, stage 3 sleep and stage 4 sleep
    b. Benzodiazepines are associated with REM rebound
    c. Tricyclic antidepressants suppress REM sleep and increase stage 4 NREM sleep
    d. Antidepressant and antipsychotic drugs increase delta activity on EEG
    e. Benzodiazepines increase beta activity and decrease alpha activity on EEG

49) Regarding pharmacological agents implicated in sexual dysfunction:
   a. Tricyclic drugs cause impaired ejaculation
   b. 5-HT agents may inhibit orgasm
   c. Dopamine agonists may lead to enhanced erection and libido
   d. Yohimbine is an α_2-adrenoreceptor antagonist, used as a treatment for both idiopathic and drug-induced male sexual dysfunction
   e. All of the above

50) A 48-year-old man with bipolar disorder had been stable on lithium monotherapy for 5 years. Over the last several months, he has become increasingly withdrawn, with fatigue and poor concentration. He has recently gained weight and complains of constipation. He has developed a dislike of cold and his voice is hoarse. On examination he has bradycardia, dry skin and slowly releasing reflexes. The most probable cause of his problems is:
   a. Lithium toxicity
   b. Hyperparathyroidism
   c. Nephrogenic diabetes insipidus
   d. Hypothyroidism
   e. Myasthenia gravis

7. Psychopharmacology: antipsychotics and organic disorders: Answers

1) e.
Mechanism of action of clozapine involves the D_4 and 5-HT receptors. In therapeutic concentrations it may occupy only 40–60% of D_2 receptors. Antipsychotic effects are usually obtained when D_2 occupancy is 60–70%.

2) d.
Haloperidol is a butyrophenone and pimozide is a diphenylbutylpiperidine.

3) c.
Blockade of α_1-adrenoreceptors causes hypotension.

4) a.
Hyperprolactinaemia is related to D_2 receptors; pimozide causes fatal dysrhythmias (torsade de pointes and prolonged QT interval).

5) d.
Benzamides are not sedative and cause insomnia.

6) e.
Risperidone is a potent antagonist of both 5-HT_2 and dopamine D_2 receptors.

7) b.
Nausea and abdominal pain are the main gastrointestinal side-effects.

8) e.
Atypical antipsychotics include substituted benzamides and 5-HT_2–D_2 receptor antagonists.

9) e.
The metabolism of aripiprazole is inhibited by fluoxetine and ketoconazole and some antivirals; plasma concentration is reduced by carbamazepine.

10) a.
Side-effects include dry mouth, urinary hesitancy and retention, constipation, reduced sweating, blurred vision and precipitation of glaucoma.

11) a.
Side-effects such as sedation and postural hypotension may occur.

12) b.
Hyperprolactinaemia is associated with galactorrhoea, amenorrhoea, low libido and sexual dysfunction.

13) d.
Priapism is a rare side-effect of clozapine.

14) d.
Occurrence of agranulocytosis is approximately 1%.

15) c.
Olanzapine is a thienobenzodiazepine and quetiapine is a dibenzothiazepine.

16) d.
Torticolis, tongue protrusion, grimacing and opisthotonus occur; reaction occurs soon after the treatment and is common in young men; anticholinergic agents control the reaction.

17) b.
Akathisia is an unpleasant feeling of physical restlessness and the need to move.

18) c.
QT prolongation is a rare side-effect of aripiprazole.

19) a.
Highly protein-bound compounds secrete less.

20) b.
Clozapine is useful for treating psychotic symptoms of Parkinsonism.

21) d.
Blockade of D_2 in the nigrostriatal pathway causes Parkinsonian side-effects of neuroleptics; it occurs in 15% of cases only.

22) e.
Parkinsonian side-effects are related to the antidopaminergic action on the basal ganglia.

23) e.
Antipsychotics except amisulpride are metabolized by the liver.

24) e.
Unlike other extra-pyramidal side-effects, tardive dyskinesia does not always remit when the drugs are stopped.

25) b.
Tardive dyskinesia occurs in only 20% of schizophrenics on long-term treatments. Anti-Parkinsonian drugs usually aggravate tardive dyskinesia.

26) e.
Tardive dyskinesia is occasionally seen in patients who have not taken antipsychotic drugs.

27) e.
Neuroleptic malignant syndrome is associated more closely with high-potency antipsychotics.

28) d.
Neuroleptic malignant syndrome is associated with combined lithium and antipsychotic treatment.

29) e.
Neuroleptic malignant syndrome treatment is symptomatic: stop the drug; cool the patient; maintain fluid balance; and treat infections.

30) d.
Fluoxetine inhibits few hepatic cytochrome P450 enzymes.

31) e.
Carbamazepine induces hepatic enzymes.

32) d.
Anticholinergic anti-Parkinsonian drugs may cause constipation.

33) e.
All the drugs listed can cause impaired glucose tolerance and weight gain.

34) e.
All these drugs have anti-adrenergic effects, which could cause sexual dysfunction. All the drugs listed could also cause hyperprolactinaemia, resulting in sexual dysfunction.

35) d.
Phenothiazine, haloperidol, quetiapine, olanzapine, risperidone and clozapine could cause SIADH.

36) a.
SSRIs, clonidine, risperidone, etc. are also used in the treatment.

37) d.
Taste disturbance is a common side-effect of bupropion.

38) e.
Dilated pupils are a feature of opioid withdrawal.

39) c.
Lofexidine is a centrally acting α_2-adrenergic antagonist.

40) c.
Total body water and lean body mass decrease.

41) c.
Donepezil is reversible, rivastigmine is non-competitive and memantine is an NMDA antagonist.

42) e.
Memantine is not an anticholinesterase; it acts through the NMDA receptor.

43) a.
Amantadine is a weak dopamine antagonist with modest anti-Parkinsonian effects.

44) b.
Hypersexuality is a rare side-effect.

45) d.
Prochlorperazine is used to treat psychosis.

46) b.
Cocaine bugs (formification) are a feature of cocaine intoxication.

47) d.
The most probable diagnosis is Wernicke's encephalopathy as he presented with the symptom triad ataxia−nystagmus−ophthalmoplegia.

48) b.
REM sleep is associated with a high level of brain activity.

49) e.
Antipsychotics and SSRIs are associated with sexual dysfunction.

50) d.
Lithium interferes with thyroid hormone production.

Further reading

British National Formulary. *BNF 57*. London: Pharmaceutical Press. Also available at: www.bnf.org/bnf.

Cookson J, Taylor D, Katona C. *Use of Drugs in Psychiatry*, 5th edn. London: Gaskell, 2002.

Gelder M, Andreasen N, Lopez-Ibor J, Geddes J. Chapter 21. In: *New Oxford Textbook of Psychiatry*, 2nd edn. Oxford: Oxford University Press, 2009.

Rosenbaum JF, Arana GW, Hyman SE, Labbate LA, Fava M. *Handbook of Psychiatric Drug Therapy*, 5th edn. Baltimore, MD: Lippincott Williams and Wilkins, 2005.

Sadock BJ, Sadock VA. Chapter 36. In: *Kaplan and Sadock's Synopsis of Psychiatry*, 10th edn. Baltimore, MD: Lippincott Williams and Wilkins, 2008.

Stahl SM. *Stahl's Essential Psychopharmacology: Neuroscientific Basis and Practical Applications*, 3rd edn. Cambridge: Cambridge University Press, 2008.

8. Clinical psychiatry 1: Questions

History and mental state examination

1) Which of the following is closest to the meaning of empathy as a psychiatric term?

   a. Keeping your feelings inside
   b. Listening to patients sympathetically
   c. Feeling sorry about the patient's problems
   d. Feeling oneself into the patient's difficulties
   e. Giving advice to patients about their problems

2) Which of the following is a closed question?

   a. Do you get headaches?
   b. How do you feel today?
   c. At what time do you wake?
   d. When did the pain start?
   e. Tell me about your problem.

3) Which of the following is not advisable while interviewing a violent patient?

   a. Checking for an alarm button
   b. Being close to the door
   c. Staying calm
   d. Getting close to the patient physically
   e. Watching out for signs of increasing anger

4) Details of a patient's childhood relationship with his/her parents is part of:

   a. History of present illness
   b. Family history
   c. Personal history
   d. Past illnesses
   e. Mental state examination

5) Which of the following best describes a patient who appears cheerful while describing sad events?

   a. Agitation
   b. Elation of mood
   c. Fluctuation of mood
   d. Incongruity of mood
   e. Depressed mood

6) Which of the following is not true about assessing risk of suicide?

   a. It is an important part of mental state examination
   b. It should be asked about in stages
   c. It should be explored in detail
   d. Is an important clinical skill to be learned
   e. It carries the risk of suggesting suicide to people who are depressed

7) A person who reports having heard his name called out while waking up from sleep is likely to have:

   a. Auditory illusions
   b. Hypnagogic hallucinations
   c. Hypnopompic hallucinations
   d. First-person auditory hallucinations
   e. Second-person auditory hallucinations

8) Serial sevens is a test of:

   a. Abstract thinking
   b. IQ
   c. Attention and concentration
   d. Short-term memory
   e. Long-term memory

9) A patient reporting that people sitting at a distance are discussing him is likely to have:

   a. Third-person hallucinations
   b. Second-person hallucinations
   c. Delusions of grandiosity
   d. Delusions of reference
   e. Thought broadcast

10) Which of the following is not an important task at the time of initial psychiatric interview?

   a. Establishing good rapport
   b. Information gathering
   c. Risk assessment
   d. Establishing a diagnosis
   e. Building treatment alliance

11) Which of the following does not fit into Bleuler's description of schizophrenia?

   a. Loosening of associations
   b. Auditory hallucinations
   c. Incongruity of affect
   d. Autism
   e. Splitting of mind

12) Which of the following is not a disorder of perception?

a. Attention
b. Illusions
c. Hallucinations
d. Pseudohallucinations
e. Misperceptions

Neurological examination

13) In a patient with spinal cord injury, which of the following does not indicate posterior column damage?

a. Positive Romberg's sign
b. Diminished tendon reflex
c. Increased muscle tone
d. Loss of vibration sense
e. Loss of proprioception

14) Which of the following is not a feature of an upper motor neuron lesion?

a. Cog-wheel rigidity
b. Up-going planters
c. Clonus
d. No muscle loss
e. Increased tendon reflexes

15) Which of the following illnesses can present with diplopia?

a. Oculomotor nerve neuropathy
b. Facial nerve neuropathy
c. Parkinson's disease
d. Huntington's disease
e. Diabetes insipidus

16) Which of the following is not a feature of normal-pressure hydrocephalus?

a. Ataxia
b. Intention tremor
c. Cognitive deficits
d. Urinary incontinence
e. Enlarged ventricles on CT brain scan

17) Which of the following conditions does not present with nystagmus?

a. Brain stem lesions
b. Cerebellar lesions
c. Frontal cortex lesions
d. Labyrinthine disease
e. Rotational stimulation

18) A patient presenting with sensory and motor deficits in the right lower limb along with clouding of consciousness is likely to have developed:

    a. Middle cerebral artery occlusion
    b. Anterior cerebral artery occlusion
    c. Posterior cerebral artery occlusion
    d. Posterior inferior cerebellar artery occlusion
    e. Interior inferior cerebellar artery occlusion

19) Which of the following structures is involved in the direct and consensual lights reflex pathway?

    a. Superior colliculus
    b. Lateral geniculate body
    c. Visual cortex
    d. Primary motor cortex
    e. Ciliary ganglion

20) Which of the following structures is most likely to be damaged in a patient presenting with left homonymous hemianopia?

    a. Left optic tract
    b. Optic chiasma
    c. Right lateral geniculate body
    d. Left medial geniculate body
    e. Visual cortex

21) Which of the following is not a cerebellar sign?

    a. Nystagmus
    b. Dysdiadochokinesia
    c. Past pointing
    d. Dysarthria
    e. Tremors at rest

22) Which of the following conditions will not be part of the differential diagnosis in a patient presenting with papilloedema?

    a. Central retinal vein thrombosis
    b. Cavernous sinus thrombosis
    c. Cranial arteritis
    d. Carotid artery occlusion
    e. Hypoparathyroidism

23) Which of the following is likely to be seen in cerebral artery occlusion?

a. Spontaneous pain
b. Ipsilateral hemianalgesia
c. Ipsilateral hemianaesthesia
d. Ipsilateral hemiplegia
e. Ipsilateral hemianopia

24) Colour vision is tested with the help of which of the following?

a. Snellen chart
b. Jensen chart
c. Ishihara chart
d. Takayashi chart
e. Wernicke chart

25) 'Tunnel vision' is characteristic of which of the following conditions?

a. Macular degeneration
b. Retinitis pigmentosa
c. Chronic glaucoma
d. Retinal detachment
e. Optic nerve atrophy

26) Which of the following is not associated with Argyll Robertson pupil?

a. Small-sized pupil
b. Irregular-shaped pupil
c. Caused by syphilis
d. Lack of sympathetic nerve supply to the pupil
e. Pupils affected bilaterally

27) Which of the following ocular muscles is not supplied by the third cranial nerves?

a. Lateral rectus
b. Medial rectus
c. Superior rectus
d. Inferior rectus
e. Inferior oblique

28) Which of the following is not true of Bell's palsy?

a. It is lower motor neuron palsy of facial nerve
b. It is usually bilateral
c. It causes difficulty in shutting eyes
d. It causes difficulty in raising eyebrows
e. It produces a loss of sense of taste

29) Which of the following statements is not true about the trigeminal nerve?

   a. It consists of motor and sensory components
   b. Motor components supply the muscles of swallowing
   c. Sensory components are responsible for general sensations to the face
   d. It is responsible for the consensual component of corneal reflex
   e. It is the motor supply to the muscles of mastication

30) While examining deep tendon reflexes, which of the following reflex and associated spinal segment pairs is incorrect?

   a. Biceps–C5 and 6
   b. Triceps–C7
   c. Supinator–C5 and 6
   d. Knee–L1 and 2
   e. Ankle–S1 and 2

31) While examining gait disturbances, which of the following pairs of gait disturbance and common cause is incorrect?

   a. Shuffling–Parkinson's disease
   b. Waddling–Muscular dystrophy
   c. Marche à petits pas–Cerebellar pathology
   d. Foot slapping–Neuropathy
   e. Drunken and wide based–Cerebellar pathology

32) Visual field defects affecting both eyes are indicative of a lesion at which of the following levels?

   a. Retinal lesions
   b. Lesions of optic nerve
   c. Lesions of optic chiasma
   d. Lesions of or behind the optic chiasma
   e. Lesions of sensory cortex

33) On fundoscopy, a patient presents with unilateral papilloedema. Which of the following conditions could be the most likely cause?

   a. Intracranial tumour
   b. Brain abscess
   c. Encephalitis
   d. Hydrocephalus
   e. Optic nerve glioma

34) A Kayser–Fleischer ring is characteristic of which of the following?

   a. Parkinson's disease
   b. Huntington's disease
   c. Wilson's disease
   d. Addison's disease
   e. Diabetes mellitus

35) A positive Romberg's sign is indicative of which of the following?

   a. Loss of proprioceptive control
   b. Loss of muscle tone
   c. Loss of motor control
   d. Loss of sensation
   e. Loss of hand–eye coordination

36) In a patient presenting with a wrist drop, which of the following nerves is most likely to be affected?

   a. Ulnar nerve
   b. Radial nerve
   c. Median nerve
   d. Musculocutaneous nerve
   e. Axillary nerve

Cognitive assessment

37) Which of the following is not a test of attention and concentration?

   a. Digit span
   b. Cognitive estimates
   c. Orientation in time and place
   d. Serial sevens
   e. Timed letter or star cancellation task

38) Which of the following is a definition of semantic memory?

   a. Memory of numbers
   b. Memory of events
   c. Memory of facts and concepts
   d. Memory of words and their meanings
   e. Memory of facts and concepts and words and their meanings

39) Episodic and semantic memory are components of which of the following memory systems?

   a. Long-term memory
   b. Short-term memory
   c. Working memory
   d. Procedural memory
   e. Conditioned reflexes

40) Which of the following cognitive functions is not attributed to frontal lobes?

   a. Abstract thinking
   b. Problem solving
   c. Planning
   d. Praxis
   e. Set shifting

41) Which of the following conditions is less likely to present with a disorder of frontal lobes?

   a. Alzheimer's disease
   b. Pick's disease
   c. Huntington's disease
   d. Parkinson's disease
   e. Wilson's disease

42) Which of the following tests is not used for frontal lobe function?

   a. Verbal fluency
   b. Digit span
   c. Cognitive estimates
   d. Proverb interpretation
   e. Motor sequencing

43) While differentiating between delirium and dementia, which of the following cognitive domains is less likely to be affected in dementia?

   a. Attention
   b. Short-term memory
   c. Episodic memory
   d. Speech
   e. Perception

44) Which of the following dementias can present with a classical mixture of cortical and sub-cortical features?

   a. Alzheimer's disease
   b. Creutzfeld–Jakob disease
   c. Lewy body dementia
   d. Huntington's disease
   e. Wilson's disease

45) Which of the following cognitive functions is not localized in the non-dominant hemisphere?

   a. Visual perceptual skills
   b. Praxis
   c. Constructional ability
   d. Melody
   e. Vigilance

46) Which of the following areas in the brain is responsible for language comprehension and production?

   a. Broca's area
   b. Wernicke's area
   c. Orbitofrontal cortex
   d. Dorsolateral frontal cortex
   e. Occipital cortex

47) Which of the following terms refers to the correct use of prepositions, pronouns, adverbs and verbs in a language?

   a. Phonology
   b. Semantic
   c. Syntax
   d. Prosody
   e. Articulation

48) Which of the following is a definition of dyslexia?

   a. Disorder of calculation
   b. Disorder of writing
   c. Disorder of reading
   d. Disorder of praxis
   e. Disorder of construction

49) A tendency to produce erroneous material to fill in the gaps on being questioned about past events is known as:

   a. Retrograde amnesia
   b. Anterograde amnesia
   c. Global amnesia
   d. Confabulation
   e. Lying

50) A patient has presented with left-sided neglect. Which of the following areas of the brain is most likely to be affected?

   a. Right parietal and prefrontal cortex
   b. Left parietal and prefrontal cortex
   c. Right orbitofrontal cortex
   d. Left orbitofrontal cortex
   e. Right basal ganglia

51) Which of the following does not apply to dressing apraxia?

   a. It is difficulty in dressing
   b. It is a disorder of the motor coordination of the upper limbs
   c. It is a disorder of visual–spatial mechanisms
   d. It may be seen in advanced dementia
   e. It may be seen in focal lesions of the right parietal cortex

52) Which of the following is not a feature of Klüver–Bucy syndrome?

a. Bilateral frontal lobe damage
b. Increased sexual drive
c. Emotional blunting
d. Passivity
e. Indiscriminate eating.

53) Which of the following is not a dominant (left) hemisphere function?

a. Spontaneous speech
b. Writing
c. Calculation
d. Construction
e. Praxis

54) In a patient in the early stage of Alzheimer's disease, which of the following tests can be used to estimate pre-morbid IQ?

a. Boston naming test
b. Graded naming test
c. National Adult Reading Test
d. Cognitive estimates
e. Raven's progressive matrices

55) Which of the following statements is true about most tests of intellectual ability?

a. Almost all are culturally fair
b. Almost all are completely free from practice effect
c. Educational level can affect performance
d. Only memory is tested
e. They are not affected by language

56) Which of the following statements is not true about the Wisconsin Card-Sorting Test?

a. It is used to study abstract behaviour
b. It is used to study set-shifting ability
c. It picks up perseveration errors
d. People with frontal lobe damage score low
e. People with subcortical dementia score normal

57) Which of the following calculation difficulties is most likely to be seen in mild-to-moderate Alzheimer's disease?

a. Difficulty in writing numbers
b. Difficulty in reading numbers
c. Difficulty in comprehending numbers
d. Difficulty in mathematical calculations
e. All of the above

8. Clinical psychiatry 1: Answers

1) d.
Empathy is a skill used in an interview to assess the patient's internal subjective state by putting oneself into his/her shoes.

2) a.
It is important to allow the patient as far as possible to describe the problem spontaneously.

3) d.
It is advisable not to approach the patient too closely and to avoid prolonged eye contact.

4) c.
Any prolonged separation from parents and the patient's reaction to it, excessive fears, etc. should be assessed.

5) d.
Although the abnormality of incongruity of affect is said to be highly characteristic of schizophrenia, different interviewers tend to disagree about its presence.

6) e.
Questioning about suicide during examination does not suggest suicide to people who have no suicidal inclination.

7) c.
Hypnapompic hallucinations occur when waking up from sleep. They are usually auditory but can be visual or tactile. They occur in normal people.

8) d.
Serial sevens is included in the Mini Mental State Examination.

9) d.
Extracampine hallucinations may also present in a similar way, when a patient experiences hallucinations outside the limits of the sensory field (concrete awareness).

10) d.
Establishing a diagnosis is not an important task in the initial psychiatric interview.

11) b.
The primary symptoms of schizophrenia are known as the four 'A's: associative disturbances; affective disturbances; autism; and ambivalence.

12) a.
Abnormal perception includes sensory distortion and false perception.

13) c.
Fine touch, pressure, vibration, position sensation, tactile discrimination, tactile localization and stereognosis are the posterior column sensations.

14) a.
Cog-wheel rigidity is not a feature of upper motor neuron lesions. In peripheral nerves, these lesions occur above the level of the anterior horn cells in the spinal cord and in cranial nerves, they occur above the level of the motor nuclei.

15) a.
The oculomotor nerve supplies the extraocular muscles except superior oblique and lateral rectus.

16) b.
Normal-pressure hydrocephalus is a treatable cause of cognitive impairment.

17) c.
The frontal cortex is associated with functions like mood, personality and executive functions and language.

18) b.
Unilateral occlusion of the anterior cerebral artery produces contralateral sensorimotor deficits mainly involving the lower extremity, but sparing the face and hands.

19) e.
Ciliary ganglion is a feature of Argyll Robertson pupil, which is seen in syphilis.

20) c.
Hemianopia is loss of half of the visual field.

21) e.
Intention tremor is seen.

22) c.
Papilloedema is seen in increased intracranial pressure.

23) a.
Ipsilateral means same side.

24) c.
The Snellen chart tests visual acuity.

25) b.
Retinitis pigmentosa is an inherited retinal degeneration.

26) d.
The loss of sympathetic fibres occurs in Horner's syndrome.

27) a.
The oculomotor nerve supplies the extraocular muscles except superior oblique and lateral rectus.

28) b.
Bell's palsy is usually unilateral.

29) b.
Trigeminal nerves supply the muscles of mastication and not of swallowing.

30) d.
Knee jerk is supplied by L3 and 4.

31) c.
Marche à petits pas is classically seen in hydrocephalus.

32) d.
Optic chiasma is the part of the brain where the optic nerves partially cross.

33) e.
Optic glioma is the most common primary neoplasm of the optic nerve.

34) c.
A Kayser–Fleischer ring reflects copper deposition in the brain.

35) a.
A positive Romberg test suggests sensory ataxia.

36) b.
Radial neuropathy typically presents with weakness of wrist dorsiflexion (i.e. wrist drop) and finger extension.

37) b.
Cognitive estimates is a test of frontal lobe functions.

38) e.
Semantic dementia is one of the main clinical variants (progressive aphasia) of frontotemporal dementia.

39) a.
There are two types of long-term memory: episodic memory and semantic memory.

40) d.
Praxis is attributed to parietal lobes.

41) a.
In Pick's disease, knife-blade atrophy is seen.

42) b.
Digit span tests attention and concentration.

43) a.
Attention and awareness are usually unaffected in dementia and delirious patients have fluctuating attention.

44) c.
Lewy body dementia presents with memory problems and Parkinsonian symptoms.

45) b.
Praxis is localized mainly in the dominant parietal lobe.

46) b.
Broca's area is located in the left posterior inferior front cortex comprising Brodmann's areas 44 and 45. Wernicke's area is on the posterior section of the superior temporal gyrus posterior part of Brodmann's area 22.

47) c.
Syntax means the assembly of strings of words into sentences using pronouns, prepositions, etc.

48) c.
Apraxia is the inability to carry out learned purposeful movements.

49) d.
Confabulation is seen in Korsakoff's psychosis.

50) a.
The right parietal and prefrontal cortex is involved in spatial attention.

51) a.
Dressing apraxia is not a motor disorder.

52) a.
The amygdala and hypothalamus are involved in Klüver–Bucy syndrome.

53) d.
Construction is a non-dominant (right) hemisphere function.

54) c.
The National Adult Reading Test (NART) is widely used as a measure of premorbid IQ of English-speaking patients with dementia.

55) c.
In most tests of intellectual ability, the subject's educational level can have a major effect on performance.

56) e.
Subjects with subcortical dementia fail on this test.

57) d.
Acalculia is associated with parietal lobe dysfunction.

Further reading

David A, Fleminger S, Kopelman M, Lovestone S, Mellers J. *Lishman's Organic Psychiatry: A Textbook of Neuropsychiatry*, 4th edn. Chichester: Wiley-Blackwell, 2009.

Gelder M, Harrison P, Cowen P. *Shorter Oxford Textbook of Psychiatry*, 5th edn. Oxford: Oxford University Press, 2006.

Hodges JR. *Cognitive Assessment for Clinicians*, 2nd edn. Oxford: Oxford University Press, 2007.

Puri B, Hall A. *Revision Notes in Psychiatry*, 2nd edn. London: Arnold/ Hodder Education, 2004.

9. Clinical psychiatry 2: Questions

Assessment, ethics and philosophy

1) Select one correct statement regarding persistent delusional disorder:
   a. Delusional disorder is associated with passivity phenomena
   b. Delusions must be present for at least 3 months for a diagnosis
   c. Depressive episodes invalidate the diagnosis
   d. Persistent delusional disorder is associated with persistent hallucinations
   e. Somatization is an important factor in persistent delusional disorder

2) Which one of the following eye signs is pathognomonic of multiple sclerosis?
   a. Argyll Robertson pupil
   b. Bilateral internuclear ophthalmoplegia
   c. Holmes–Adie pupil
   d. Horner's syndrome
   e. Kayser–Fleischer ring

3) Regarding apraxia, which of the following statements is false?
   a. Motor system and sensorium should be sufficiently intact
   b. Constructional apraxia can be tested by asking the patient to draw simple figures
   c. Dressing apraxia is tested by asking the patient to put on some of his/her clothes
   d. Ideomotor apraxia can be tested by increasingly complicated tasks to command
   e. None of the above

4) Which of the following is false?
   a. Atopognosia is failure to identify letters written on skin
   b. Astereognosis is failure to identify three-dimensional form
   c. Finger agnosia is failure to identify which finger is touched
   d. Anosognosia is failure to identify functional deficits caused by disease
   e. Agnosia is inability to understand significance of sensory stimuli

5) Which of the following is not an interviewer-rated scale?
   a. Hamilton Rating Scale for Depression
   b. Montgomery–Åsberg Depression Rating Scale
   c. Yale–Brown Obsessive Compulsive Scale
   d. Beck Depression Inventory
   e. Hamilton Anxiety Scale

6) Which of the following statements is true?

   a. The Yale–Brown Obsessive Compulsive Scale is a seven-point scale for obsessive compulsive disorder
   b. The Brief Psychiatric Rating Scale has 10 items scored on a seven-point scale
   c. The Hamilton Rating Scale for Depression measures symptoms of depression rather than the severity
   d. The General Health Questionnaire has been primarily designed for diagnosis in primary care
   e. The Hamilton Anxiety Scale should not be used to rate anxiety in patients with other disorders

7) Regarding reliability of an instrument, which of the following is false?

   a. Interrater reliability measures degree of agreement between different raters
   b. Test–retest reliability describes degree of correlation between two identical assessments at different times
   c. Split-half reliability signifies the external consistency of a test
   d. Intrarater reliability measures degree of agreement by the same rater at different times
   e. The index of interrater reliability is kappa

8) In relation to psychometric tests, which of the following is false?

   a. Validity measures the degree to which a test can be replicated
   b. Sensitivity is the degree to which a test measures true positives
   c. A test with high specificity has a low type I error rate
   d. A positive result in a high-specificity test rules in the disease
   e. Negative predictive value is the proportion of patients with negative test results who are correctly diagnosed

9) In Alzheimer's dementia, all of the following symptoms can be seen, except:

   a. Long-term memory loss
   b. Depression
   c. Disorders of language and praxis
   d. Impairment of consciousness
   e. Persecutory delusion

10) Gerstmann's syndrome includes:

   a. Right-to-left disorientation
   b. Acalculia
   c. Dysgraphaesthesia
   d. Finger agnosia
   e. Dysgraphia

11) In Wernicke–Korsakoff's syndrome, all of the following are true, except:

    a. Anterograde amnesia is a main feature of the syndrome
    b. Hallucinations rule out Korsakoff's syndrome
    c. Vision problems include double vision and drooping of the eyelid
    d. Confabulation is very characteristic of the syndrome
    e. It is caused by thiamine deficiency

12) All of the following are true regarding pseudohallucinations, except:

    a. They are a form of imagery
    b. They are experienced as located in external space but recognized as unreal
    c. They are not diagnostic
    d. They are experienced within the mind
    e. They cannot be dismissed by an effort of will

13) All of the following are false, except:

    a. Eidetic imagery cannot be intense and detailed
    b. Perception can be terminated by an effort of will
    c. Pareidolia is a type of imagery
    d. Imagery is the awareness of the percept that has arisen from the sense organs
    e. A healthy person cannot distinguish between images and percepts

14) Regarding hallucinations, which of the following is false:

    a. They can occur in healthy individuals
    b. They cannot be terminated at will
    c. They can occur after sensory deprivation
    d. They are diagnostic of psychotic disorder
    e. They can occur in seizures

15) Which of the following is true regarding hallucinations:

    a. Hallucinatory voices are sometimes called phonemes
    b. Hallucinations of dwarf figures are called extracampine hallucinations
    c. In second-person hallucination, voices refer to the patient as he or she
    d. Elementary hallucination refers to experiences such as seeing faces and scenes
    e. Gedankenlautwerden is when voices repeat the thoughts immediately after the patient has thought them

16) Select one correct statement from the following:

   a. Écho de la pensée is when voices seem to speak the patient's thoughts as he/she is thinking them
   b. Olfactory and gustatory hallucinations are frequently experienced together
   c. Hypnopompic hallucinations occur at the point of falling asleep
   d. Haptic hallucination is a type of olfactory hallucination
   e. Reflex hallucination is common in schizophrenia

17) All of the following are types of loosening of association, except:

   a. Verbigeration
   b. Vorbeireden
   c. Word salad
   d. Knight's move
   e. Over-inclusion

18) All of the following are true, except:

   a. Autochthonous delusions are primary delusions
   b. Delusions are systematized when delusions accumulate and become a complicated delusional system
   c. Change of mood before a delusion is called Wahnstimmung
   d. Capgras syndrome is a delusion in which a familiar person is replaced by an impostor
   e. Delusional mood is a type of delusional memory

19) Regarding depersonalization, all of the following are true, except:

   a. The person feels unreal, detached from his/her own experience
   b. It is a pleasant experience
   c. The experience begins abruptly and lasts only a few minutes in healthy people
   d. It is not diagnostic
   e. It is experienced quite commonly as a transient phenomenon by healthy adults

20) All of the following are true regarding motor symptoms, except:

   a. Tics are regular repeated movements involving a group of muscles
   b. Mannerisms are repeated movements that appear to have some functional significance
   c. Posturing is the adoption of unusual bodily postures continuously for a long time
   d. Stereotypes are repeated movements that are regular and without obvious significance
   e. Psychological pillow is a type of waxy flexibility

21) The following are all disorders of body image, except:

    a. Coenestopathic state
    b. Mitgehen
    c. Phantom limb
    d. Hemiasomatognosia
    e. Reduplication phenomenon

22) Regarding memory, which of the following is false?

    a. Semantic memory is concerned with factual information
    b. Episodic memory is memory for experiences
    c. Procedural memory is also called explicit memory
    d. Prospective memory is also concerned with actions to be carried out in the near future
    e. Working memory usually holds information for 15–20 seconds

23) All of the following are true, except:

    a. Jamais vu is failure to recognize events that have been encountered before
    b. Déjà vu is the conviction that an event has occurred when in fact it is novel
    c. Retrograde amnesia is inability to recall events before onset of unconsciousness
    d. In amnestic disorder, people can recall remote events but not events from a few minutes before
    e. Anterograde amnesia is a disorder of recognition

24) Which of the following is true in types of impaired level of consciousness?

    a. Oneiroid state is a dream-like state in sleep
    b. Torpor is a state of impaired consciousness with no evidence of slow thinking
    c. Twilight state is a prolonged oneiroid state
    d. In stupor, reflexes are abnormal
    e. The patient does not resist attempts to open a closed eye in stupor

25) In the Mini Mental State Examination:

    a. Orientation to time, place and person are assessed
    b. Constructional praxis is checked by clock drawing
    c. Left-to-right orientation is assessed
    d. Spelling 'world' backwards assesses concentration
    e. Abstract reasoning is assessed by interpretation of proverbs

26) Which of the following is false?

 a. Language disorders point to left hemisphere in right-handed people
 b. Dysarthria is difficulty in the production of speech by the speech organs
 c. Dysphasia is partial failure of the language function of cortical origin
 d. Receptive dysphasia suggests a posterior lesion
 e. Language disorder with mainly visual dysphasia suggests an anterior lesion

27) Regarding scales, which of the following is false?

 a. The Mini Mental State Examination has 30 items
 b. The Hamilton Anxiety Scale has 21 items
 c. The Montgomery–Åsberg Depression Rating Scale has 10 items
 d. The Brief Psychiatric Rating Scale has 16 items
 e. The Yale–Brown Obsessive Compulsive Scale has 10 items

28) Regarding anxiety, which of the following is false?

 a. Somatic anxiety is where the subject has increased tension and fearful apprehension
 b. Anxiety symptoms are part of normal healthy experience
 c. A moderate amount of anxiety can optimize performance
 d. Anxiety symptoms may occur only episodically in panic attacks
 e. Anxiety symptoms may not have an identifiable stimulus

29) Which of the following is not a first-rank symptom?

 a. Thought insertion
 b. Thought echo
 c. Thought withdrawal
 d. Thought broadcasting
 e. Thought block

30) In the Glasgow Coma Scale (GCS), which of the following is false?

 a. The total score is 15
 b. The maximum score for verbal response is 6
 c. A GCS score of 8 or less correlates with severe brain injury
 d. A person able to speak only inappropriate words scores 3 in verbal response
 e. A person able to flex only to pain scores 3 in motor response

31) Which of the following statements is false?

  a. The Wisconsin Card-Sorting Task is used to assess frontal lobe functioning
  b. The go/no-go test is used as part of the frontal assessment battery
  c. Astereognosia is seen in non-dominant parietal lobe lesion
  d. Gerstmann's syndrome is caused by a lesion of the dominant parietal lobe
  e. The maximum score in the Mini Mental State Examination for assessing orientation is 10

32) All of the following physical signs could be suggestive of the corresponding physical illnesses, except:

  a. Hamster face—bulimia nervosa
  b. Lanugo hair—anorexia nervosa
  c. Goose flesh—opiate withdrawal
  d. Broad-based gait—cerebellar disease
  e. Argyll Robertson pupil—Wilson's disease

33) All of the following can be described as features of schizophrenia, except:

  a. Ambitendency
  b. Asyndesis
  c. Blunting of affect
  d. Broca's dysphasia
  e. Derailment

34) Narcolepsy consists of all of the following, except:

  a. Catalepsy
  b. Excessive daytime sleepiness
  c. Sleep paralysis
  d. Sudden loss of muscle tone
  e. Hypnagogic hallucinations

35) First-rank symptoms include all of the following, except:

  a. Somatic passivity
  b. Passivity of volition
  c. Paucity of speech
  d. Passivity of impulse
  e. Passivity of affect

36) Which of the following is false?

  a. Othello syndrome is delusional jealousy
  b. Ekbom's syndrome is delusion of infestation
  c. De Clérambault's syndrome is delusion of love
  d. Capgras syndrome is delusional misidentification
  e. Fregoli's syndrome is delusion of reference

37) All of the following are synonyms, except:

  a. Entgleiten–Derailment
  b. Erotomania–Delusion of love
  c. Ey syndrome–Othello syndrome
  d. Écho de la pensée–Thought echo
  e. Gedankenlautwerden–Thought echo

38) All of the following are features of Wernicke's encephalopathy, except:

  a. Ophthalmoplegia
  b. Nystagmus
  c. Ataxia
  d. Acute confusional state
  e. It is caused mainly by vitamin B12 deficiency

39) Regarding normal-pressure hydrocephalus, all of the following are true, except:

  a. Dementia is irreversible
  b. Gait ataxia is present
  c. Urinary incontinence usually appears later
  d. Dilation of cerebral ventricles is present
  e. 24-hour intracranial pressure monitoring shows a typical 'beta' pattern

40) In Parkinson's disease, all of the following are seen, except:

  a. Cog-wheel rigidity
  b. Resting tremor
  c. Bradykinesia
  d. Negative glabellar tap
  e. Autonomic instability

41) Which of the following is not part of the widely propounded principles of moral philosophy and ethics proposed by Beauchamp and Childress (1994)?

  a. Autonomy
  b. Beneficence
  c. Non-maleficence
  d. Logical analysis
  e. Justice

42) Regarding principles of confidentiality, all of the following are true, except:

a. Wherever possible, identifiable data should be used
b. Disclosure should be done only after consent
c. Children over a stated age (usually 16) should enjoy the same rights as adults
d. Disclosure of information should be kept to a minimum
e. Effective measures should be taken to protect personal information

43) Medical treatment may be given in all of the following situations, except:

a. When the patient has offered written consent
b. In an emergency
c. When it is considered in the best interest of an unconscious patient
d. When it is for a patient with capacity who has refused consent
e. When the patient has given implied consent

44) Under the Mental Capacity Act 2007, a patient is stated to have capacity if he/she is able to do all of the following, except:

a. Comprehend the information
b. Believe the information
c. Retain the information
d. Make an informed choice
e. Communicate his/her decision

45) Legal criteria for assessing testamentary capacity include all of the following, except:

a. Whether a testator understands what a will is and what its consequences are
b. Whether he/she knows the nature and extent of the property
c. Whether he/she knows the names of close relatives and can assess their claims to the property
d. Whether he/she has suffered any mental illness in the past
e. Whether he/she is free from an abnormal state of mind that might distort feelings or judgements relevant to making the will

46) Regarding driving after an illness, the Driver and Vehicle Licensing Agency regulations include all of the following, except:

a. One year off driving after a solitary fit
b. 4 weeks off driving after the event if the person has loss of consciousness likely to be unexplained syncope and low risk of recurrence
c. Must not drive for at least one month after a cerebrovascular disease
d. Must not drive after a diagnosis of dementia
e. 3 months off driving after the person has been well and stable after an acute psychotic disorder, compliant with treatment and receives a favourable specialist report

47) According to the Driver and Vehicle Licensing Agency, a person suffering from schizophrenia or other chronic psychosis can restart driving after an acute episode if he/she satisfies all of the following conditions, except:

a. Stable behaviour for at least 3 months
b. Adequately compliant with treatment
c. Free from adverse effects of medication that would impair driving
d. Subject to a favourable specialist report
e. Should have full insight

48) Which of the following is false regarding General Medical Council guidelines for informing the Driver and Vehicle Licensing Agency?

a. The DVLA is legally responsible for deciding if a patient is medically unfit to drive
b. The doctor should request the patient to inform the DVLA if the patient has a condition which impairs the ability to drive
c. The doctor has to inform the DVLA without the patient's knowledge of any condition which could impair the ability to drive
d. If the patient does not accept the diagnosis or effect of the condition on ability to drive, the doctor should suggest a second opinion
e. If the patient continues to drive when not fit to do so, the doctor should make every reasonable effort to persuade the patient to stop

49) Confidentiality may be broken in all the following situations, except:

a. To assist in the prevention or detection of a crime
b. If a close friend wants to know the diagnosis against the patient's wishes
c. If the general public are at serious risk
d. If the patient continues to drive when unfit to do so and against medical advice
e. For notification of a known or suspected communicable disease

50) In relation to the Mental Health Act 1983, which of the following is incorrect?

a. Section 5(4) is holding power for a maximum of 72 hours
b. Section 2 provides authority for a patient to be detained in hospital for assessment for a maximum of 28 days
c. Section 136 is for police to take a person in a public place who is considered to be mentally disordered to a 'place of safety'
d. Section 3 is a treatment order initially for a maximum period of 6 months
e. Section 2 cannot be renewed or extended after 28 days

9. Clinical psychiatry 2: Answers

1) b.
According to the ICD-10 classification, delusion constitutes the most conspicuous or the only clinical characteristic and must have been present for at least 3 months.

2) b.
A pathognomic feature of multiple sclerosis is bilateral internuclear ophthalmoplegia.

3) e.
All are true.

4) a.
Atopognosia is failure to know the position of an object on the skin while agraphognosia is failure to identify letters or numbers written on the skin.

5) d.
The Beck Depression Inventory is client rated.

6) e.
Yale–Brown is a four-point scale for 10 symptoms. The Brief Psychiatric Rating Scale has 16 items scored on seven-point scale. Hamilton measures severity rather than the symptoms. GHQ is a screening questionnaire used in primary care.

7) c.
Split-half reliability signifies internal consistency.

8) a.
Validity measures the extent to which a test measures what it is designed to measure.

9) d.
Impairment of consciousness is seen in delirium rather than dementia.

10) c.
Gerstmann's syndrome consists of all the other four symptoms.

11) b.
Korsakoff's psychosis consists of hallucinations and is a late stage of Wernicke's encephalopathy.

12) a.
Pseudohallucinations resemble imagery but, unlike imagery, they cannot be dismissed by an effort of will.

13) c.
Eidetic memory is visual imagery that is so intense and detailed that it has a 'photographic' quality. Perception can be attended to or ignored but cannot be terminated by an effort of will. Imagery is awareness of the percept that has arisen from the mind and not the sense organs. Images lack the sense of reality by which healthy people distinguish them from percepts.

14) d.
Hallucination is not diagnostic.

15) a.
Hallucinations of dwarf figures are called Lilliputian hallucinations. Voices refer to the patient as he or she in third-person hallucination, while in second-person hallucination voices talk to the patient. As the name explains, elementary hallucination refers to flashes of light, bangs, whistles, etc. Gedankenlautwerden is voices that seem to speak the patient's thoughts as he/she is thinking them, while écho de la pensée is voices that seem to repeat the thoughts immediately after the patient has thought them.

16) b.
Hypnagogic hallucinations occur at point of sleep and hypnopompic at time of getting up. Haptic hallucinations are tactile hallucinations. Reflex hallucination is a rare condition.

17) e.
Verbigeration is speech reduced to senseless repetition of sounds, words or phrases. Vorbeireden is talking past the point. Word salad is severe verbigeration. Knight's move is jumping from one topic to another. Over-inclusion is a disorder of thought form but not part of loosening of association.

18) e.
Delusional mood is different from delusional memory. In delusional memory, past events are processed with new significance.

19) b.
Depersonalization is reported to be a very unpleasant experience.

20) a.
Tics are irregular repeated movements.

21) b.
Mitgehen is abnormal body movement in which the patient's body movement can be initiated with the slightest pressure.

22) c.
Procedural memory is implicit memory, in which patients cannot explain the steps for a procedure but can do it.

23) e.
Anterograde amnesia is a disorder of memory.

24) c.
Oneiroid state occurs when the patient is not sleeping. Torpor occurs with slow thinking and narrowed range of perception. In stupor, reflexes are normal; usually the eyes are open and if they are closed the patient will resist any attempt to open them.

25) d.
Orientation to person is not assessed. Constructional praxis is checked by an interlocking pentagon. Abstract reasoning and left-to-right orientation are not assessed in the MMSE.

26) e.
Language disorder with mainly visual dysphasia suggests a posterior lesion.

27) b.
In the Hamilton Anxiety Scale, 13 items are rated, using five-point scales.

28) a.
In psychic anxiety the subject has increased tension and fearful apprehension, while in somatic anxiety the patient has bodily sensations of palpitation and sweating.

29) e.
Thought block is not a Schneiderian first-rank symptom.

30) b.
In the Glasgow Coma Scale, the best eye, verbal and motor response scores are 4, 5 and 6 respectively.

31) c.
Astereognosis is failure to recognize the feel of objects with the eyes closed. It is seen in dominant parietal lobe lesions.

32) e.
Argyll Robertson pupil is seen in neurosyphilis.

33) d.
Broca's dysphasia is not a feature of schizophrenia.

34) a.
This is a common question. It is cataplexy and not catalepsy that is seen in narcolepsy.

35) c.
First-rank symptoms do not include paucity of speech.

36) e.
Fregoli's syndrome is a type of delusional misidentification. The patient believes strangers have been replaced by familiar people.

37) a.
Entgleisen is a synonym for derailment. Entgleiten is a synonym for thought blocking.

38) e.
Wernicke's encephalopathy is caused by vitamin B1 deficiency and not B12. The other four are the classical tetrad in Wernicke's.

39) a.
Dementia is potentially reversible if treated promptly.

40) d.
In Parkinson's disease there is usually positive glabellar tap.

41) d.
The other four form the principles of moral philosophy and ethics.

Beauchamp TL, Childress CF. *Principles of Biomedical Ethics*, 4th edn. Oxford: Oxford University Press, 1994.

42) a.
Non-identifiable data should be used.

43) d.
Consent is needed in a patient with capacity.

44) b.
In the latest Act, the 'believe' part has been omitted.

45) d.
Testamentary capacity does not deal with past history.

46) d.
People with mild dementia may drive after notifying the DVLA if they have been found fit to drive, though they may have to undergo a special extended driving test.

47) e.
The DVLA checks fitness to drive.

48) c.
The patient should be notified or informed before the doctor informs the DVLA if necessary.

49) b.
Patient consent is needed if no risk issues are identified.

50) a.
Section 5(4) is about nurses holding power for 6 hours.

Further reading

David A, Fleminger S, Kopelman M, Lovestone S, Mellers J. *Lishman's Organic Psychiatry: A Textbook of Neuropsychiatry*, 4th edn. Chichester: Wiley-Blackwell, 2009.

Gelder M, Harrison P, Cowen P. *Shorter Oxford Textbook of Psychiatry*, 5th edn. Oxford: Oxford University Press, 2006.

ICD-10: *The ICD-10 Classification of Mental and Behavioural Disorders: Clinical Descriptions and Diagnostic Guidelines*. Geneva: World Health Organization, 1990.

Puri B, Hall A. *Revision Notes in Psychiatry*, 2nd edn. London: Arnold/Hodder Education, 2004.

Sadock BJ, Sadock VA. *Kaplan and Sadock's Synopsis of Psychiatry*, 10th edn. Baltimore, MD: Lippincott Williams and Wilkins, 2008.

10. Clinical psychiatry 3: Questions

History, classification and stigma

1) Which of the following biological treatments was not an empirical discovery?

   a. General paralysis by malaria therapy
   b. Schizophrenia by insulin coma
   c. Depression by malaria therapy
   d. Schizophrenia by chemically induced seizures
   e. Depression by electroconvulsive therapy

2) The term 'démence précoce' was introduced by:

   a. Schneider
   b. Bleuler
   c. Morel
   d. Kraepelin
   e. Jaspers

3) Bleuler's four 'A's exclude:

   a. Ambivalence
   b. Blunting of affect
   c. Loosening of associations
   d. Autism
   e. Altruism

4) Schneider's first-rank symptoms do not include:

   a. Thought block
   b. Thought withdrawal
   c. Delusional perception
   d. Somatic passivity
   e. Third-person hallucinations

5) Which of the following is false in the axial system of DSM-IV?

   a. Axis 1 provides information about major mental disorder
   b. Axis 2 provides information about personality disorder
   c. Axis 3 provides information about mental retardation
   d. Axis 4 is used to describe environmental factors
   e. Axis 5 is a rating scale called Global Assessment of Function

6) The term 'catatonia' was coined by:

a. Goffman
b. Kraepelin
c. Schneider
d. Kahlbaum
e. Morel

7) The term 'hebephrenia' was coined by:

a. Morel
b. Bleuler
c. Kraepelin
d. Schneider
e. Hecker

8) Which of the following features is not part of the type 1 syndrome described by Crow:

a. Good response to neuroleptics
b. Abnormal cerebral structures
c. Presumed dysfunction in the dopamine system
d. Predominantly positive symptoms
e. Good prognosis

9) Erikson's stages of psychosocial development do not include:

a. Initiative versus guilt
b. Identity versus role confusion
c. Intimacy versus isolation
d. Autonomy versus inferiority
e. Integrity versus despair

10) Which of the following statements about Freud's psychosexual stages of development is false?

a. The anal stage is characterized by orderliness
b. The oral stage is characterized by envy
c. The phallic stage is characterized by competitiveness
d. The oral stage is characterized by dependence
e. The phallic stage is characterized by obsessionality

11) In which stage of Piaget's model does a child understand that the same volume of water can be contained in a tall jar as in a broad jar?

a. Sensorimotor stage
b. Preoperational stage
c. Concrete operational stage
d. Formal operational stage
e. None of the above

12) Gestalt principles do not include:

    a. Figure–ground similarity
    b. Continuity
    c. Closure
    d. Simplicity
    e. Proximity

13) According to Maslow's hierarchy of needs:

    a. Physiological or physical needs can be achieved after safety needs
    b. Aesthetic needs can be achieved after cognitive needs
    c. Esteem comes before belonging and love
    d. Self-actualization can be achieved before aesthetic needs
    e. Esteem is achieved after cognitive needs

14) Which of the following is not a part of the social power described by French and Raven?

    a. Reward
    b. Authority
    c. Immediacy
    d. Expertise
    e. Referential

15) Which of the following is false?

    a. Task completion is poor in laissez-faire leadership
    b. Urgent tasks are better done by autocratic leadership
    c. There is more liking within the group in democratic leadership
    d. There is good interaction with the leader in laissez-faire leadership
    e. In democratic leadership, the group can continue in the absence of the leader

16) According to Sigmund Freud's earliest model:

    a. Conscious involves primary process
    b. Preconscious content can be brought into consciousness through selective attention
    c. Unconscious is governed by the reality principle
    d. Preconscious involves the pleasure principle
    e. Information is readily available from the unconscious

17) Which of the following is false regarding Freud's structural model?

a. Id is the unconscious reserve of impulses
b. Ego is the part that mediates with the external world
c. Superego is the person's values, morals and ethics derived from parents
d. Id functions at all three levels of conscious, preconscious and unconscious
e. Superego develops in the second year of life

18) Find the odd one out:

a. Carl Jung: animus and anima
b. Melanie Klein: paranoid-schizoid position
c. Anna Freud: individual psychology
d. Donald Winnicott: good-enough mother
e. Friedrich Perls: Gestalt therapy

19) Which of the following is not an autosomal recessive disorder?

a. Niemann–Pick disease
b. Tay–Sachs disease
c. Hunter syndrome
d. Hurler syndrome
e. Lesch–Nyhan syndrome

20) Which of the following is true?

a. External locus of control is associated with poor response to stress
b. Internal locus relates to a feeling that life is externally controlled and determined
c. People with type A personality are very relaxed
d. No conscious recollection or temporal awareness is needed in implicit retrieval
e. Secondary reinforcement is not based on prior learning

21) Which of the following is true?

a. Impairment refers to a pathological deficit
b. Disability is the stable persistent limitation of physical or psychological function
c. Handicap refers to continuing social dysfunction
d. None of the above
e. All of the above

22) Regarding the ICD-10 classification system, which of the following is false?

    a. It is hierarchical
    b. It is multiaxial
    c. It is dimensional
    d. It is available in different versions
    e. It is available in all widely spoken languages

23) Regarding DSM-IV, which is true?

    a. It is published by the American Psychiatric Association
    b. Different versions are available
    c. It is available in widely spoken languages
    d. It is a single-axis system
    e. The criteria do not include social consequences of impairment

24) An elderly man in the postoperative ward has been presenting with fluctuating cognition for the last 24 hours. Staff also reported that he has been seen to respond to hallucinations. The most likely diagnosis is:

    a. Alzheimer's dementia
    b. Lewy body dementia
    c. Delirium
    d. Vascular dementia
    e. Pseudodementia

25) Regarding Rett syndrome, which of the following is false?

    a. It is reported only in girls
    b. It usually involves abnormal early development
    c. Onset begins between 7 and 24 months of age
    d. There is loss of acquired hand skills and speech
    e. There is deceleration in head growth

26) Asperger's syndrome is:

    a. A specific developmental disorder of speech and language
    b. A mixed specific developmental disorder
    c. A specific developmental disorder of scholastic skills
    d. A pervasive developmental disorder
    e. None of the above

27) Which of the following is true regarding ICD-10 classification?

   a. Lewy body dementia is not classified in the dementia category
   b. Delirium superimposed on dementia is classified under the organic amnestic syndrome not induced by alcohol and other psychoactive substances
   c. Dementia beginning before the age of 55 years is classified as dementia in Alzheimer's disease with early onset
   d. CT scan is diagnostic in Alzheimer's dementia
   e. Typically symptoms should be present for at least 1 year for confident clinical diagnosis of dementia

28) According to ICD-10, all of the following should be present for a diagnosis of dependence syndrome, except:

   a. Symptoms should be present at some time during the previous year
   b. Evidence of tolerance
   c. Difficulty in controlling substance-taking behaviour
   d. Sense of compulsion
   e. The desire to take the particular substance is absent currently

29) For a diagnosis of catatonic schizophrenia, predominant behaviours need to include all the following according to ICD-10, except:

   a. Stupor
   b. Posturing
   c. Excitement
   d. Negativism
   e. Depression

30) Which of the following is false regarding post-schizophrenic depression?

   a. The patient should have had schizophrenia in the last year
   b. No symptoms of schizophrenia should be present now
   c. Depressive symptoms should be prominent and distressing
   d. Depressive symptoms should have been present for at least 2 weeks
   e. It is classified under schizophrenia, schizotypal and delusional disorders

31) In ICD-10, psychotic disorder as a result of mental and behaviour disorders due to use of alcohol includes all of the following, except:

   a. Alcoholic hallucinosis
   b. Alcoholic jealousy
   c. Alcoholic dementia
   d. Alcoholic paranoia
   e. Alcoholic psychosis not otherwise specified

32) Regarding phobias, which of the following is false?

a. Claustrophobia is a fear of closed spaces
b. Arachnophobia is a fear of spiders
c. Acrophobia is a fear of open spaces
d. Hydrophobia is a fear of water
e. Cynophobia is a fear of dogs

33) Which of the following is true according to ICD-10 diagnostic criteria?

a. In mania, symptoms should have been present for at least 2 weeks
b. In hypomania, symptoms should have been present for at least several days
c. In depression, symptoms should have been present for at least I week
d. In acute schizophrenia-like psychotic disorder, symptoms last for more than I month
e. In delusional disorder, symptoms must have been present for at least I month

34) Regarding diagnosis of anorexia nervosa, which of the following is false?

a. Body weight is maintained at least 15% below that expected
b. Weight loss is self-induced by avoidance of 'fattening food'
c. There is body-image distortion
d. A widespread endocrine disorder involving the hypothalamo-pituitary-gonadal axis is seen
e. If onset is prepubertal, pubertal changes are arrested that are irreversible

35) Which of the following is true?

a. Ganser syndrome is a type of dissociative disorder
b. Nightmare is a type of sleep terror
c. Somatoform disorder is a type of somatization disorder
d. Hypochondriacal disorder is the same as somatization disorder
e. Neurasthenia is a type of somatoform disorder

36) Which of the following does not come under 'Other anxiety disorder' in ICD-10?

a. Panic disorder
b. Post-traumatic stress disorder
c. Generalized anxiety disorder
d. Episodic paroxysmal anxiety
e. Mixed anxiety and depressive disorder

37) All of the following are classified into 'Schizophrenia, schizotypal and delusional disorder' in ICD-10, except:

    a. Delusional disorder
    b. Simple schizophrenia
    c. Schizotypal disorder
    d. Schizoid personality disorder
    e. Residual schizophrenia

38) Which of the following is false regarding the symptom and the associated personality disorder?

    a. Inappropriate seductiveness–Histrionic
    b. Feeling of emptiness–Borderline
    c. Callous concern for feeling of others–Dissocial
    d. Recurrent suspicions–Schizoid
    e. Perfectionist–Anankastic

39) All of the following are types of 'Other somatoform disorders' in ICD-10, except:

    a. Psychogenic backache
    b. Psychogenic torticollis
    c. Globus hystericus
    d. Psychogenic dysmenorrhoea
    e. Teeth-grinding

40) Schizotypal disorder consists of all of the following, except:

    a. Inappropriate affect
    b. Poor rapport with others
    c. Odd or eccentric behaviour
    d. Suspiciousness or paranoid ideas
    e. Prominent hallucinations that are dominant

41) All of the following culture-bound syndromes are correctly matched with their corresponding areas, except:

    a. Amok–Malaysia
    b. Ashanti–West Africa
    c. Koro–Malaysia
    d. Dhat–India
    e. Brain fag–Mexico

42) Regarding ghost sickness, which of the following is false?

    a. It is a preoccupation with death
    b. Subjects may say they have been 'bewitched'
    c. Subjects complain of nightmares
    d. It is seen in native Africans
    e. Subjects may have a sense of suffocation

43) Amok consists of all of the following, except:

    a. It involves sudden, unprovoked, random acts of violence
    b. It may be preceded by a period of depression
    c. The subject always has delusions or another thought disorder
    d. The subject is amnesic about the violent acts
    e. The subject may commit suicide later

44) All of the following are true regarding latah, except:

    a. It is an exaggerated startle reaction
    b. It occurs predominantly in elderly women
    c. It occurs following sudden fright/trauma
    d. It is trance-like behaviour
    e. It may be a symptom of disease

45) Which of the following is true of piblokto?

    a. It is usually seen in Arctic men
    b. It is also known as Antarctic hysteria
    c. It may be preceded by convulsions or coma
    d. There is never any associated amnesia of the event
    e. It occurs following the actual loss of someone or something

46) According to Littlewood and Lipsedge (1987), culture-bound syndromes share all of the following characteristics, except:

    a. They occur in people who are 'powerful' and socially very accepted
    b. They usually occur in young men or women
    c. They are usually dramatic, and the individual is unaware or not responsible
    d. They have a symbolic cultural significance
    e. They show a typical triphasic pattern

47) All of the following are true regarding ashanti, except:

    a. It is seen usually in women
    b. It consists of two subtypes
    c. It may follow a difficult childbirth or death of the child
    d. It is also known as brain fag
    e. A frenzied guilt and fear subtype may follow physical illness and fever

48) Which of the following is true regarding wendigo?

   a. It is seen in East Africans
   b. It is a delusion of being transformed into a giant monster
   c. The subject feels very happy
   d. The subject is respected by other people on being transformed
   e. It is a very common syndrome

49) All of the following are true regarding susto, except:

   a. It is seen in elderly people
   b. It is prevalent in Peru, Mexico and other Latin American countries
   c. It is a belief that the soul has been or will be stolen from the body
   d. It usually follows an acute stressor
   e. It is characterized by significant body weight loss and sleep disturbance

50) Which of the following is seen usually in men?

   a. Sar
   b. Pibloko
   c. Latah
   d. Ashanti
   e. Amok

1) c.
Malaria therapy was for general paralysis.

2) c.
Bénédict Morel, a French psychiatrist, introduced the term 'démence précoce'. Kraepelin later made it into the dementia precox.

3) e.
Altruism is not one of the four 'A's.

4) a.
Thought block is not a first-rank symptom.

5) c.
Axis 2 provides information about personality disorder and mental retardation, while axis 3 provides information about general medical condition.

6) d.
Kahlbaum described catatonia in 1874.

7) e.
Hecker described hebephrenia.

8) b.
Structural abnormalities are seen in type 2 syndrome.

9) d.
Erikson's stage 4 of psychosocial development is industry versus inferiority. Autonomy versus shame and doubt is stage 2.

10) e.
Anal stage relates to obsessionality. According to Freud, incomplete resolution of the stages leads to pathological traits in adulthood.

11) c.
Development of logical thought and laws of conservation are attained by the concrete operational stage.

12) a.
Figure–ground differentiation is included in Gestalt's principles. It is ability to differentiate the figure from the background in a picture.

13) b.
Maslow's hierarchy of needs consists of physiological/physical, safety, social, esteem, cognitive, aesthetic, and self-actualization needs.

14) c.
Coercion is the fifth type of social power.

15) d.
Interaction with the leader is poor in laissez-faire leadership.

16) b.
Preconscious and conscious involve a secondary process and are governed by the reality principle. Unconscious entails primary process thinking and is governed by the pleasure principle.

17) d.
This theory was initiated by Cade in 1949 but it was too controversial at that time. It later became popular in the 1960s.

18) c.
Anna Freud was involved in describing defense mechanisms. Alfred Adler was the founder of individual psychology.

19) e.
Lesch–Nyhan syndrome is an X-linked recessive disorder.

20) a.
External locus relates to the feeling that life is externally controlled. Type A personalities are very anxious.

21) e.
All three statements are true.

22) c.
ICD-10 is a categorical classification.

23) a.
DSM-IV is available only in a single version for both clinical and research purposes. It is available only in English and is a multi-axial system.

24) c.
Delirium is the most usual presentation in a postoperative ward.

25) b.
Rett syndrome features normal early development.

26) d.
Asperger's syndrome is a pervasive developmental disorder.

27) a.
ICD-10 classifies only dementia in Parkinson's disease.

28) e.
A strong desire or sense of compulsion to take the substance should be present for a diagnosis of dependence syndrome.

29) e.
Depression is not a feature of catatonia.

30) b.
Some schizophrenic symptoms are still present in post-schizophrenic depression.

31) c.
Alcoholic dementia is not classified in psychotic disorder, but is classified in residual and late-onset psychotic disorder.

32) c.
Acrophobia is fear of heights.

33) b.
In mania, symptoms should have been present for at least 1 week. In depression, symptoms should have been present for at least 2 weeks. In acute schizophrenia-psychotic disorder, symptoms last for less than 1 month. In delusional disorder, symptoms must have been present for at least 3 months.

34) e.
With recovery, puberty is often completed normally.

35) a.
Somatization disorder is a type of somatoform disorder. In somatization emphasis is on symptoms, while in hypochondriacal disorder emphasis is on the presence of a disease. Neurasthenia comes under 'other neurotic disorder'.

36) b.
PTSD comes under 'Reaction to severe stress and adjustment disorders'.

37) d.
Schizoid personality disorder comes under 'Specific personality disorder'.

38) d.
Recurrent suspicion is seen commonly in 'Paranoid personality disorder'.

39) a.
Psychogenic backache comes under 'Persistent somatoform pain disorder'.

40) e.
There is no dominant or typical disturbance in schizotypal disorder.

41) e.
Brain fag is seen in West African students.

42) d.
Ghost sickness is seen in Native Americans.

43) c.
Amok is a sudden random attack of violence that may be preceded by a period of depression or anxiety.

44) b.
Latah is predominantly seen in young girls.

45) e.
Piblokto is also known as 'Arctic hysteria' and is seen in polar Eskimo women.

46) a.
Culture-bound syndromes are usually seen in 'powerless' and socially neglected young men or women.

Littlewood R, Lipsedge M. *Aliens and Alienists: Ethnic Minorities and Psychiatry*. Harmondsworth: Penguin, 1987.

47) d.
Brain fag is a syndrome seen in West African students.

48) b.
Windigo is seen in Native Americans. It is a very uncommon syndrome.

49) a.
Susto is seen in children and adults.

50) e.
Amok is seen in Malayan males.

Further reading

Diagnostic and Statistical Manual of Mental Disorders, 4th edn (DSM-IV). Arlington, VA: American Psychiatric Association, 1994.

Gelder M, Harrison P, Cowen P. *Shorter Oxford Textbook of Psychiatry*, 5th edn. Oxford: Oxford University Press, 2006.

ICD-10: The ICD-10 Classification of Mental and Behavioural Disorders: Clinical Descriptions and Diagnostic Guidelines. Geneva: World Health Organization, 1990.

Puri B, Hall A. *Revision Notes in Psychiatry*, 2nd edn. London: Arnold/Hodder Education, 2004.

Sadock BJ, Sadock VA. *Kaplan and Sadock's Synopsis of Psychiatry*, 10th edn. Baltimore, MD: Lippincott Williams and Wilkins, 2008.

11. Clinical psychiatry 4: Questions

Organic and psychotic disorders

1) The most frequent symptom of schizophrenia is:

    a. Auditory hallucinations
    b. Lack of insight
    c. Delusional mood
    d. Delusions of persecution
    e. Flatness of affect

2) Schneiderian first-rank symptoms include all of the following, except:

    a. Delusional perception
    b. Thoughts spoken aloud
    c. Paranoid delusion
    d. Thought insertion, withdrawal and broadcasting
    e. Somatic passivity

3) Which of the following is true of schizophrenia?

    a. First-rank symptoms are pathognomonic of schizophrenia
    b. The ICD-10 general criteria for schizophrenia are based on Schneider's first-rank symptoms
    c. The ICD-10 general criteria for schizophrenia require the presence of symptoms and signs lasting for at least 6 months
    d. The prevalence of schizophrenia varies widely in different countries
    e. The DSM-IV-TR diagnostic criteria for schizophrenia require the onset of symptoms between the ages of 15 and 45

4) All of the following are true, except:

    a. The onset of schizophrenia characteristically occurs between the ages of 15 and 45
    b. Well controlled evidence indicates that a specific family pattern plays a causative role in the development of schizophrenia
    c. Schizophrenia is equally prevalent in men and women
    d. Onset of schizophrenia is earlier in men than women
    e. People who develop schizophrenia are more likely to have been born in the winter and early spring

5) Which of the following is true of people suffering from schizophrenia?

    a. A higher mortality rate from accidents and natural causes is observed
    b. Men have lower social class distribution than their fathers
    c. Men are more likely to drift into inner-city areas
    d. 10–15% commit suicide
    e. All of the above

6) Which of the following statements is correct regarding research evidence in the aetiology of schizophrenia?

    a. A positive correlation between high pre-treatment central nervous system concentration of homovanillic acid and the severity of psychotic symptoms is observed
    b. Agonistic activity at the serotonin 5-HT_2 receptor reduces psychotic symptoms
    c. There is an increase in the size of the limbic area in patients with schizophrenia
    d. The changes in regional brain volume in patients with schizophrenia show a clear association with gender
    e. Movement disorders unrelated to antipsychotic drug treatment have been more associated with late-onset illness

7) Which of the following is the most frequent behavioural abnormality associated with schizophrenia?

    a. Social withdrawal
    b. Neglect of appearance
    c. Threats of violence
    d. Suicide attempts
    e. Sexually unusual behaviour

8) Regarding clinical features of schizophrenia, all of the following are true, except:

    a. In acute schizophrenia, orientation is usually impaired
    b. Depressive symptoms in schizophrenia may be a response to recovery of insight
    c. About 50% of patients with acute schizophrenia experience acute depressive symptomatology
    d. Water intoxication is associated with schizophrenia
    e. The social background of the patient may affect content of symptoms

9) Which of the following types of hallucinations occur in schizophrenia?

a. Visual
b. Tactile
c. Olfactory
d. Gustatory
e. All of the above

10) All of the following are regarded as aetiologically related to schizophrenia, except:

a. Schizotypal personality disorder
b. Schizoid personality disorder
c. Winter birth
d. Prenatal exposure to influenza
e. Obstetric complications

11) A 30-year-old man was brought to the hospital for his ninth admission, the first one being at the age of 16. He was observed to have a child-like quality to his speech and manner and he walks with an exaggerated hip movement. His speech is incoherent and his behaviour is disorganized. He also had some fleeting and fragmentary delusions and hallucinations. The most probable diagnosis is:

a. Paranoid schizophrenia
b. Hebephrenic schizophrenia
c. Catatonic schizophrenia
d. Undifferentiated schizophrenia
e. Simple schizophrenia

12) Regarding subtypes of schizophrenia as classified in ICD-10, all of the following are true, except:

a. In paranoid schizophrenia, disturbances of affect and catatonic symptoms are relatively inconspicuous
b. Hebephrenia should normally be diagnosed only in adolescents or young adults
c. Episodes of violent excitement may be a striking feature of catatonic schizophrenia
d. A depressive state with florid and prominent schizophrenic symptoms is characteristic of post-schizophrenic depression
e. Chronic undifferentiated schizophrenia is classified under residual schizophrenia

13) Regarding prognosis of schizophrenia, all of the following are true, except:

    a. Increased relapse rate is associated with a high expressed emotion in the family

    b. Family history of affective disorder is a predictor of good prognosis

    c. Later onset is a good prognostic indicator

    d. High educational attainment is protective against a high risk of suicide

    e. Akathisia increases risk of suicide

14) Which of the following statements about delusional disorder is true?

    a. Erotomanic type is a subtype in DSM-IV

    b. It is more common in men

    c. Mean age of onset is earlier in females

    d. It is more common when there is an increased family history of schizophrenia

    e. Marked personality changes occur

15) A 64-year-old man admitted on the ward has delusions that all his wealth has gone. He also believes that his organs are decaying and that people hate him because of the smell of his rotten body parts. The most probable diagnosis is:

    a. De Clérambault's syndrome

    b. Cotard's syndrome

    c. Capgras syndrome

    d. Fregoli's syndrome

    e. Folie à deux

16) A 45-year-old woman on the ward believes that her daughter has been replaced by a double. The most probable diagnosis is:

    a. De Clérambault's syndrome

    b. Cotard's syndrome

    c. Capgras syndrome

    d. Fregoli's syndrome

    e. Folie à deux

17) Regarding delusional syndromes, which of the following is true?

    a. Erotomania is more common in males

    b. Capgras syndrome is more common in males

    c. Pathological jealousy is more common in males

    d. Induced psychosis (folie à deux) involves members of the same family only

    e. The primary cause of Capgras syndrome is always an organic brain dysfunction

18) In ICD-10:

a. Schizotypal disorder and schizoid personality disorder are classified separately

b. The presence of occasional or transitory auditory hallucinations, particularly in elderly patients, rules out the diagnosis of delusional disorder

c. Delusional dysmorphophobia is classified under 'Other schizophrenia'

d. If acute and transient psychotic disorder persists for more than 72 hours, a change in diagnosis is necessary

e. Mood-incongruent psychotic symptoms in affective disorders by themselves justify a diagnosis of schizoaffective disorder

19) Disorientation is commonly associated with:

a. Acute and transient psychotic disorder

b. Organic delusional disorder

c. Delirium tremens

d. Korsakoff's psychosis

e. Alcoholic hallucinosis

20) All of the following are associated with acute intoxication from cannabinoids, except:

a. Temporal slowing

b. Auditory, visual or tactile illusions

c. Depersonalization and derealization

d. Nystagmus

e. Conjunctival injection

21) According to ICD-10, a diagnosis of substance dependence syndrome can be made if all of the following are present, except:

a. Psychological withdrawal state

b. A sense of compulsion to take the substance

c. Evidence of tolerance

d. Preoccupation with substance use

e. Persistent substance use despite clear evidence of harmful consequences

22) Features of delirium include:

a. Disorganization of the sleep–wake cycle

b. Psychomotor retardation and perseveration

c. Visual hallucinations

d. Depersonalization and derealization

e. All of the above

23) All of the following are causes of delirium, except:

    a. Catatonic schizophrenia
    b. Wernicke's encephalopathy
    c. Cushing's syndrome
    d. Head injury
    e. Sleep deprivation

24) Which of the following is true of schizophrenia-like states in elderly people?

    a. They can be aetiologically associated with sensory deprivation
    b. They are more common in males
    c. They are mostly associated with a family history of schizophrenia
    d. They are characteristically associated with visual hallucinations
    e. They respond well to antipsychotics, with remission of symptoms in 90% of cases

25) Regarding the relationship between schizophrenia and affective disorder, all of the following are true, except:

    a. At least one-third of schizophrenics have depressive symptoms
    b. There is an increased occurrence of affective disorder in family members of schizophrenics
    c. Bipolar disorder is more common in families of schizoaffective disorder patients than those of schizophrenia patients
    d. Bipolar disorder is more common in male relatives of schizophrenics
    e. Unipolar disorder is more common in female relatives of schizophrenics

26) Delirium tremens:

    a. Carries a significant risk of mortality
    b. Lasts 3–4 days
    c. Has symptoms that characteristically are worse at night
    d. Is associated with dilation of pupils and prolonged insomnia
    e. All of the above

27) Chronic alcohol misuse:

    a. Causes frontal lobe dysfunction
    b. Causes medial thalamic lesions leading to amnesia
    c. Causes up to a six-fold increase in the suicide rate
    d. Is associated with erectile and ejaculatory dysfunction
    e. All of the above

28) All of the following are true about alcohol dependence, except:

a. It aggregates in families
b. It may be mediated by dopamine release in mesolimbic pathways
c. It is increasingly observed in antisocial personality disorder
d. It is more common in Asians with decreased function of aldehyde dehydrogenase
e. It is associated with increased blood pressure

29) Pathological jealousy occurs in:

a. Paranoid schizophrenia
b. Depression
c. Alcoholism
d. Dementia
e. All of the above

30) All of the following are true about narcolepsy, except:

a. It usually begins in adolescence
b. It is more frequent in females
c. Sleep paralysis and hypnagogic hallucinations occur in 75% of patients
d. Cataplexy occurs in most cases
e. There is a family history in one-third of patients

31) Which of the following is true of transient global amnesia?

a. It commonly occurs in adolescents and young adults
b. It occurs as sudden onset of global amnesia
c. It is associated with localized perfusion abnormalities in the brain, observed on functional imaging
d. It is usually associated with abnormalities on neurological examination
e. The patient usually recovers, with amnesia of the period affected, but recurrence is common

32) Klüver–Bucy syndrome includes all of the following, except:

a. Hyperorality
b. Over-attention to external stimuli
c. Agnosia
d. Hyposexuality
e. Loss of fear

33) All of the following are common symptoms of temporal lobe epilepsy, except:

a. Olfactory hallucinations
b. Déjà vu
c. Micropsia
d. Pareidolic illusions
e. Auditory hallucinations

34) Which of the following is true of pseudodementia?

    a. It is most common in elderly depressed patients
    b. 'Don't know' responses and poor involvement on neuropsychological tests are characteristic
    c. It can be caused by conversion disorder
    d. When it is caused by a factitious disorder, a source of secondary gain may be apparent
    e. All of the above

35) All of the following are true of frontotemporal dementia, except:

    a. It is more common in young-onset dementias
    b. Behavioural disturbance includes apathy
    c. Early memory impairment is characteristic
    d. Language disturbances are frequent
    e. When caused by Pick's disease, knife-blade atrophy is common

36) Clinical manifestations of idiopathic Parkinson's disease include all of the following, except:

    a. Intention tremor
    b. Bradykinesia
    c. Mania
    d. Sexual disorders
    e. REM sleep behaviour disorder

37) Which of the following are characteristic of Huntington's disease?

    a. Onset occurs early in adolescence
    b. It is autonomic recessive
    c. Purposeless fidgeting choreiform movements occur, which the patient may attempt to disguise
    d. It has low rates of affective disorders
    e. Predictive genetic testing is not currently available

38) Subdural haematoma:

    a. Usually lacks a history of head injury
    b. Is often associated with hemiparesis and oculomotor signs
    c. Can cause a dementia-like picture
    d. Surgical evacuation may reverse the symptoms
    e. All of the above

39) Regarding prion diseases, all of the following are true, except:

   a. Creutzfeldt–Jakob disease is the most common
   b. Sporadic disease accounts for less than 50% of cases
   c. Kuru is transmitted by ritual cannibalism
   d. Gerstmann–Straussler–Scheinker syndrome is an autosomal dominantly inherited prion disease
   e. They are caused by abnormal fibrillar prion glycoprotein deposition in the brain

40) All of the following statements about Creutzfeldt–Jakob disease (CJD) are correct, except:

   a. Sporadic CJD affects both sexes equally
   b. Sporadic CJD presents typically between 60 and 65 years
   c. Sporadic CJD is usually heralded by cognitive decline
   d. Variant CJD is linked with bovine spongiform encephalopathy
   e. It often progresses to death within several years

41) A 73-year-old man has been referred to the memory clinic with a history of memory problems over the last 6 months. He presents with a broad-based small-stepped gait with difficulty in initiation, and slowing in response. His wife reported that he has developed urinary incontinence recently. The most probable diagnosis is:

   a. Creutzfeldt–Jakob disease
   b. Lewy body dementia
   c. Dementia pugilistica
   d. Normal-pressure hydrocephalus
   e. Subdural haematoma

42) A 58-year-old man presented to the memory assessment service with a history of personality changes over the last 12 months with progressive impairment in his language function. He was observed to have paralysis of the extra-ocular muscles, dysarthria, cervical and truncal dystonia and ataxia. The most probable diagnosis is:

   a. Creutzfeldt–Jakob disease
   b. Huntington's disease
   c. Progressive supranuclear palsy
   d. Wernicke's encephalopathy
   e. Multiple sclerosis

43) Which of the following is true of alcohol?
   a. It produces its effects in the brain mainly through action on NMDA receptors
   b. At higher levels it can cause death secondary to respiratory depression and aspiration
   c. Its use is associated with increased REM sleep and stage 4 sleep
   d. It is associated with elevation of γ-GT in a minor proportion of people with alcohol-related disorders
   e. Carbohydrate-deficient transferrin is identified as a biomarker for chronic alcoholism with high sensitivity and low specificity

44) Foetal alcohol syndrome includes:
   a. Craniofacial malformations
   b. Small stature
   c. Low birth weight
   d. Mental retardation and over-activity
   e. All of the above

45) Postnatal blues:
   a. Are characterized by tearfulness, emotional lability and confusion
   b. Occur in 50% of women
   c. Peak at the third to fifth days postpartum
   d. Are aetiologically linked to progesterone withdrawal after delivery
   e. All of the above

46) Puerperal psychosis is characterized by all of the following, except:
   a. Gradual onset within the first 2 months of childbirth
   b. No detectable cognitive impairment
   c. Rapid fluctuations in mental state
   d. Marked restlessness, fear and insomnia
   e. Delusions and hallucinations

47) All of the following are correct about erectile dysfunction, except:
   a. It is organic in about 90% of cases
   b. It can be caused by Peyronie's disease
   c. Hyperprolactinaemia secondary to alcoholism can be a cause
   d. Naltrexone therapy improves impotence of apparent non-organic cause
   e. Alpha-adrenergic blockers are not usually associated with erectile dysfunction but may cause ejaculatory failure

48) Which of the following is true of night terrors:

 a. They occur during stage 3 and 4 sleep
 b. They usually occur 1 or 2 hours after sleep starts
 c. There is little recall the following morning
 d. Enuresis may occur during an episode
 e. All of the above

49) Which of the following is true of delirium?

 a. It affects 10–25% of over-65-year-olds admitted to medical wards
 b. It is more marked in conditions with poor illumination
 c. Visual misinterpretations are common
 d. Mortality can be up to 30–40% because of the underlying condition
 e. All of the above

50) All of the following are true of late-onset psychosis, except:

 a. It is more common in females
 b. 40–45% of cases present with Schneiderian first-rank symptoms
 c. 80% of cases present with visual hallucinations
 d. Sensory impairment is associated with development of paranoid symptoms
 e. About a quarter of patients show full response to treatment

1) b.
Lack of insight is a symptom in 97% of cases of schizophrenia, auditory hallucinations in 74%.

2) c.
First-rank symptoms occur in other psychoses; they are highly suggestive of schizophrenia but not characteristic of it.

3) b.
ICD-10 general criteria require symptoms for 1 month and DSM-IV for 6 months. The incidence and prevalence are roughly equal in all countries: incidence is 0.17–0.54 per 1000 population and prevalence 1.4–4.6 per 100 population at risk.

4) b.
Bateson's double-bind theory, Lidz's schisms and skewed families, Wynne's pseudomutual and pseudohostile family theory and expressed emotion theories try to explain family factors in the aetiology, but there is no good evidence.

5) e.
These are all features of the social drift theory of schizophrenia developed by Goldberg and Morrison (1963).

Goldberg EM, Morrison SL. Shizophrenia and social class. *Br J Psychiatry* 1963; **109**: 785–802.

6) a.
$5-HT_2$ antagonism reduces psychosis; there is a decrease in the size of the limbic area; movement disorders are more associated with early-onset illness.

7) a.
Social withdrawal occurs in 74% of cases of schizophrenia, neglect of appearance in 30%, sexually unusual behaviour in 8% and suicide attempts in 4%.

8) a.
In acute schizophrenia, orientation is usually normal, but it is recognized that generalized deficits in cognitive function occur.

9) e.
Auditory hallucination is the most frequent one. All other types are reported only rarely.

10) b.
Among schizotypal criteria, eccentricity, affect constriction and excessive social anxiety are linked to schizophrenia.

11) b.
The onset of hebephrenic schizophrenia (disorganized type in DSM-IV) is usually before 25 years of age.

12) d.
Either positive or negative symptoms must be present but they should not dominate the clinical picture. If these symptoms are florid and prominent, the diagnosis should remain of the appropriate schizophrenia subtype.

13) d.
High educational attainment increases the risk.

14) a.
There is an equal sex ratio or a slightly higher prevalence in females; the mean age of onset is 35 in men, 45 in women; it is more common when there is an increased family history of psychiatric problems; personality is preserved.

15) b.
Nihilistic delusions occur.

16) c.
Capgras syndrome is the delusion that a close relative has been replaced by an identical-looking impostor.

17) c.
Erotomania is also known as de Clérambault's syndrome.

18) a.
Delusional dysmorphophobia is classified under 'Other persistent delusional disorders'; acute and transient psychotic disorder develops in less than 2 weeks.

19) c.
In delirium tremens, major withdrawal (hallucinations) occurs 10–72 hours after the last drink. The signs and symptoms include visual and

auditory hallucinations, whole body tremor, vomiting, diaphoresis and hypertension.

20) d.
Nystagmus occurs in acute intoxication with alcohol.

21) a.
A physiological withdrawal state is necessary.

22) e.
Other features of delirium include impairment of immediate recall and recent memory, and disorientation in time, place or person.

23) a.
In catatonic schizophrenia, a dreamlike (oneiroid) state occurs, with vivid scenic hallucinations, but it is not delirium.

24) a.
The female:male ratio is 7:1; the most common hallucination is auditory; 50–75% of patients respond to antipsychotics, with full or partial remission.

25) c.
Bipolar disorder is equal in both.

26) e.
Despite appropriate treatment, the current mortality for patients with delirium tremens ranges from 5 to 15%. Mortality was as high as 35% prior to the era of intensive care and advanced pharmacotherapy. The most common conditions leading to death in these patients are respiratory failure and cardiac arrhythmias.

27) e.
Chronic alcohol misuse is associated with alcoholic dementia, personality deterioration, mood disorder, suicidal behaviour, impaired psychosexual function, pathological jealousy and alcoholic hallucinosis.

28) d.
Decreased function of aldehyde dehydrogenase causes an unpleasant reaction and reduces alcohol misuse.

29) e.
Disorders associated with pathological jealousy are schizophrenia, mood disorder, organic disorder, substance misuse (including alcohol) and personality disorder.

30) c.

Sleep paralysis and hypnagogic hallucinations occur in 25% of patients.

31) c.

Localized perfusion abnormalities in the brain occur in middle and later life with isolated anterograde amnesia, and recurrence is rare.

32) d.

Hypersexuality is a feature of Klüver–Bucy syndrome.

33) d.

Pareidolic illusions occur in normal people; temporal lobe epilepsy is also provoked by psychomimetic drugs (images are seen from shapes).

34) e.

Although pseudodementia commonly occurs in depressed elderly patients, it is important to understand that depression can feature early in the course of dementia as well.

35) c.

Relatively preserved memory early on is characteristic of frontotemporal dementia.

36) a.

Resting tremor is a clinical manifestation in idiopathic Parkinson's disease.

37) c.

Huntington's disease occurs typically in middle age; it is autosomal dominant with complete penetrance; it features higher rates of depression, bipolar disorder and schizophrenia; genetic testing for the causative mutation (DNA triplet repeat coding for glutamine) is now widely available.

38) e.

Acute subdural haematoma (SDH – a collection of blood over the surface of the brain) is the most common type of traumatic intracranial haematoma, occurring in 24% of patients who present comatose. SDHs are usually caused by trauma but can be spontaneous or caused by a procedure such as lumbar puncture. Anticoagulation, such as with heparin or warfarin, may be a contributing factor.

39) b.

Prion diseases or transmissible spongiform encephalopathies (TSEs) are a family of rare progressive neurodegenerative disorders that affect both humans and animals. Human prion diseases are Creutzfeldt–Jakob disease (CJD), variant Creutzfeldt–Jakob disease (vCJD), Gerstmann–Straussler–Scheinker syndrome, fatal familial insomnia and kuru.

40) e.

Creutzfeldt–Jakob disease often progresses to death within 6 months.

41) d.

In normal-pressure hydrocephalus, the presence of hippocampal atrophy indicates associated Alzheimer's disease, with a poor response to shunting.

42) c.

Progressive supranuclear palsy (PSP) is a rare degenerative disease of the brain. The disease impairs movements and balance. Many people with PSP also experience changes in mood, behaviour and personality.

43) b.

No single molecular target has been identified to mediate the effects of alcohol. Its use is associated with decreased REM and stage 4 sleep; γ-GT is elevated in 80% of people with alcohol-related disorders; carbohydrate-deficient transferrin is identified as a biomarker for chronic alcoholism with high sensitivity and low specificity.

44) e.

Intrauterine exposure to alcohol results in foetal alcohol syndrome.

45) e.

Postnatal blues are more frequent among primigravida women.

46) a.

Puerperal psychosis is characterized by abrupt onset, within the first 2 weeks of childbirth.

47) a.

Erectile dysfunction is organic in about 50% of cases.

48) e.

Night terror disorder is sometimes familial, and begins and ends in childhood, though it occasionally persists into adult life.

49) e.

In patients who are admitted with delirium, mortality rates are 10–26%.

50) c.

Some hallucinatory experiences can be present in up to 80% of cases, but auditory hallucinations are most common.

Further reading

Gelder M, Harrison P, Cowen P. *Shorter Oxford Textbook of Psychiatry*, 5th edn. Oxford: Oxford University Press, 2006.

ICD-10: The ICD-10 Classification of Mental and Behavioural Disorders: Clinical Descriptions and Diagnostic Guidelines. Geneva: World Health Organization, 1990.

Puri B, Hall A. *Revision Notes in Psychiatry*, 2nd edn. London: Arnold/Hodder Education, 2004.

Sadock BJ, Sadock VA. *Kaplan and Sadock's Synopsis of Psychiatry*, 10th edn. Baltimore, MD: Lippincott Williams and Wilkins, 2008.

12. Clinical psychiatry 5: Questions

Affective, neurotic and personality disorders

1) The use of lithium was first initiated by:
   a. Kraepelin
   b. Cade
   c. Kahlbaum
   d. Pritchard
   e. Henderson

2) Hypomania is a disorder characterized by all of the following, except:
   a. Persistent elevation of mood
   b. Decreased need for sleep
   c. Increased sexual energy
   d. Overfamiliarity
   e. Severe disruption of work and symptoms that lead to social rejection

3) All of the following statements are true about classification of affective disorders in ICD-10, except:
   a. It allows for the diagnosis of single first episodes of hypomania without the overall diagnosis of bipolar disorder
   b. It requires a single episode of mania with psychotic symptoms to be classified as bipolar disease
   c. Two or more episodes of hypomania or mania without depressive episodes should be classified as bipolar disorder
   d. To make a diagnosis of mania, the mood change must be prominent and sustained for at least 1 week, unless it is severe enough to require hospital admission
   e. In a second episode of affective disorder, if manic and depressive symptoms are prominent most of the time during a 2-week period, a diagnosis of bipolar disorder, with current episode mixed, could be made

4) All of the following statements are true about classification of depressive episode in ICD-10, except:
   a. A fifth character in the coding may be used to specify the presence or absence of a somatic syndrome in depression
   b. The presence or absence of the somatic syndrome is not specified for severe depressive episode
   c. To make a diagnosis, the depressive episode should last for 2 weeks
   d. To make a diagnosis of severe depressive episode with psychotic symptoms, the hallucinations and delusions must be mood congruent
   e. In recurrent depressive disorder, brief episodes of mild hypomanic-type symptoms occur, especially precipitated by antidepressants

5) All of the following statements are true about depression, except:

a. Learned helplessness is described as an important cognitive symptom of depression in ICD-10
b. Dysthymia is a chronic, less severe depression and ICD-10 and DSM-IV require a duration of at least 2 years to diagnose this condition
c. Development of depression in dysthymia is known as double depression
d. Masked depression is more common in the undeveloped world
e. In seasonal affective disorder, depressive episodes commence in the autumn or winter months and end in the spring or summer

6) Which of the following statements is false?

a. Childbirth can cause mania
b. 10% of people with an initial episode of depression develop mania later
c. Depression is more common in females in all age groups
d. The average age of onset of bipolar disorder is around the mid-20s
e. Bipolar disorder is more common in upper social classes

7) Which of the following may be more common in depression in old age?

a. Hypochondriachal preoccupations
b. Depressive pseudodementia
c. Psychomotor retardation or agitation
d. Behavioural disturbances like shoplifting
e. All of the above

8) Regarding affective disorders in elderly people, all of the following are true, except:

a. The Geriatric Depression Scale is helpful in the assessment as it focuses entirely on physical symptoms of depression rather than cognitive symptoms
b. Depressed patients with ischaemic brain lesions have more vascular risk factors and less family history of mood disorders than those without
c. Hypo- and hyperthyroidism can present as depression
d. The age of onset of manic episode is bimodally distributed, with peaks at 37 and 73 years
e. Late-onset mania cases appear to have less genetic loading than younger-onset cases

9) Which of the following is true of rapid cycling bipolar disorder?

a. It is characterized by two or more episodes of affective disorders within 12 months
b. It is more common in men
c. It responds well to lithium
d. Concomitant hypothyroidism is common
e. 50% of cases are induced by antidepressants

10) In DSM-IV:

    a. The presence of a single episode of hypomania or mania is sufficient to meet the criteria for bipolar affective disorder

    b. Bipolar disorder is separated into bipolar I and bipolar II

    c. The diagnosis of bipolar II is intended to indicate the importance of detecting mild hypomanic episodes

    d. Antidepressant-induced mania/hypomania is not included in the diagnosis of bipolar I or bipolar II

    e. All of the above

11) Which of the following statements is true regarding the epidemiology of bipolar and unipolar (major depression)?

    a. Lifetime risk of bipolar disorder is higher than unipolar disorder

    b. Lifetime risk of an affective illness is higher in first-degree relatives of patients with unipolar illness than in first degree relatives of patients with bipolar disorder

    c. Both bipolar and unipolar disorders occur more commonly in females

    d. Average age of onset is higher in bipolar disorder than unipolar disorder

    e. All of the above

12) Which of the following is aetiologically linked to mood disorders?

    a. Chromosomes 4, 12 and 18

    b. Cyclothymic personality

    c. Childhood physical and sexual abuse

    d. Overprotective parental style

    e. All of the above

13) Which of the following includes endocrine causes of depression?

    a. Cushing's syndrome

    b. Addison's disease

    c. Hypothyroidism

    d. Hyperparathyroidism

    e. All of the above

14) Suicide:

    a. Suicide is more common in women

    b. Suicide is more common in people aged less than 45

    c. Suicide rates are highest in winter

    d. Suicide rates fall in times of war and natural calamities

    e. Suicide rates are lowest in social classes I and V

15) Regarding psychiatric problems and suicide, all of the following statements are true, except:

a. 90% of people who commit suicide suffer from a psychiatric disorder
b. 90% of psychiatric patients who commit suicide suffer from depression
c. 10% of the mortality in schizophrenia is from suicide
d. 5% of psychiatric patients who commit suicide suffer from schizophrenia
e. 15% of the mortality in alcoholism is from suicide

16) All of the following are true about deliberate self-harm (DSH), except:

a. Following an act of DSH, the risk of committing suicide in the first year is approximately 100 times higher than that in the general population
b. It is more common in females
c. It is more common in people below the age of 35 years
d. The highest rates are in upper social classes
e. 90% of cases involve deliberate self-poisoning

17) The Tuckman and Youngman scale for assessment of risk factors for subsequent completion of suicide awards one point to each of the following criteria, except:

a. Age above 35
b. Unemployed
c. Living alone
d. Recent medical treatment
e. Violent attempt

18) The term 'neurasthenia' was introduced by:

a. Beard
b. Hecker
c. Freud
d. Tyrer
e. Paykel

19) Regarding the classification of neurotic, stress-related and somato-form disorders in ICD-10, all of the following statements are true, except:

a. Although the term 'neurotic disorders' has been retained, the concept of neurosis has not been used as a major principle of classification
b. For the diagnosis of acute stress reaction, the symptoms should occur within 1 hour of exposure to the stressor and disappear within 2–3 days
c. For the diagnosis of adjustment disorders, the symptoms should occur within 1 month of exposure to a psychological stressor
d. Post-traumatic stress disorder is described as an adjustment disorder classified under F43.2
e. The category 'Reaction to severe stress and adjustment disorders' differs from others in that it includes symptoms and causative influences

20) All of the following are true of post-traumatic stress disorder (PTSD), except:

a. It arises within 6 months of exposure to the traumatic event
b. Autonomic disturbances are present
c. About 50% of people exposed to a potentially traumatic event develop the condition
d. Female gender is a vulnerability factor
e. Viewing the dead body of a relative after a disaster is predictive of lower PTSD

21) The DSM-IV diagnosis of acute stress reaction requires all of the following symptoms, except:

a. A sense of numbing or detachment
b. Increased awareness of surroundings
c. Derealization
d. Depersonalization
e. Dissociative amnesia

22) Which of the following is true of grief?

a. In normal grief, the second stage can last up to 6 months
b. Depressive symptoms are a frequent component of normal grief
c. Grief can be considered abnormal if the first stage has not occurred by 2 weeks after the death
d. Grief can be considered abnormal when the symptoms meet the criteria for a depressive disorder
e. All of the above

23) Regarding phobic anxiety disorders, all of the following conditions are more common in females, except:

a. Agoraphobia
b. Social phobia
c. Animal phobia
d. Miscellaneous specific phobias
e. None of the above

24) In all types of phobias, high rates of comorbidity are found with:

a. Depression
b. Alcohol abuse
c. Drug abuse
d. Obsessive compulsive disorder
e. All of the above

25) All of the following are thought to be aetiologically linked to phobic anxiety disorders, except:

   a. Fear of castration in Freud's psychoanalytic theory
   b. Pavlovian classical conditioning
   c. Operant conditioning
   d. Seligman's preparedness theory
   e. Chromosome 18

26) All of the following are true of agoraphobia, except:

   a. The term was first used by Westphal
   b. ICD-10 describes panic disorder as a frequent feature of both present and past episodes
   c. According to DSM-IV, cases with more than 4 panic attacks within 4 weeks are classified as panic disorder with secondary agoraphobic symptoms
   d. Usually onset is in childhood
   e. 80% of agoraphobics are never symptom free after 5 years of follow-up

27) Which of the following is true of panic disorder?

   a. It requires several attacks within 1 month for diagnosis in ICD-10
   b. Onset is rare after the age of 40
   c. It is twice as common in females
   d. Mitral valve prolapse occurs in 40% of cases
   e. All of the above

28) Early-onset generalized anxiety disorder is more likely to be associated with all of the following, except:

   a. Female gender
   b. History of childhood fears
   c. Marital or sexual disturbance
   d. Stressful life events
   e. None of the above

29) Which of the following is true of obsessive compulsive disorder?

   a. It is very common in children
   b. It is more common in females
   c. Patients perform well on tests of shifting set
   d. It is frequent in families of probands with Tourette's syndrome, regardless of whether the proband has OCD
   e. It has a good prognosis in males with early onset

30) All of the following are favourable prognostic factors in obsessive compulsive disorder, except:

    a. Predominance of phobic ruminative ideas
    b. Absence of compulsions
    c. No childhood symptoms
    d. Symptoms involving the need for symmetry and exactness
    e. Absence of family history of OCD

31) Common themes shared by dissociative or conversion disorders include a partial or complete loss of:

    a. The normal integration between memories of the past
    b. Awareness of identity
    c. Awareness of immediate sensations
    d. Control of bodily movements
    e. All of the above

32) All of the following are true of dissociative disorders, except:

    a. They tend to remit after a few weeks or months, when associated with a traumatic life event
    b. More chronic disorders are associated with symptoms of paralysis and anaesthesias
    c. More chronic disorders are associated with insoluble problems or interpersonal difficulties
    d. Patients present with symptoms representing their concept of how a physical illness would be manifest
    e. They include malingering

33) Which of the following is true of dissociative amnesia?

    a. It is more common in elderly people
    b. It includes memory impairment caused by fatigue
    c. It rarely lasts more than 2 days
    d. The patient usually recovers partially
    e. Recurrence is common

34) Which of the following is not characteristic of dissociative fugue?

    a. It may include a purposeful journey away from home
    b. A new identity may be assumed
    c. Self-care and social interaction are impaired
    d. It lasts for hours to days
    e. Recovery is abrupt and complete

35) Which of the following is not a principal feature of Ganser syndrome?

a. Approximate answers
b. Clouding of consciousness
c. Somatic conversion
d. Hallucinations
e. Subsequent amnesia

36) Which of the following is true of multiple personality disorder?

a. It is not included in ICD-10
b. Two or more personalities are evident at any time
c. The dominant personality has access to memories of the other
d. It includes Couvade's syndrome, which usually occurs in pregnant women
e. It is viewed in psychoanalysis as a result of childhood trauma beginning before the age of 5

37) Which of the following is true of somatization disorder?

a. It is characterized by multiple recurrent somatic complaints for at least 1 year
b. It usually begins after the age of 30
c. It was first described by Briquet
d. It is four times more common in women than men
e. It occurs commonly with alexithymia

38) Body dysmorphic disorder:

a. Is separately classified in DSM-IV
b. Is a subgroup of hypochondriasis in ICD-10
c. Was first described as dymorphophobia by Morselli
d. May involve complaints about any part of the body
e. All of the above

39) ICD-10 categories of personality disorder include all of the following, except:

a. Schizotypal
b. Paranoid
c. Dissocial
d. Anancastic
e. Dependent

40) Which of the following subtypes of personality disorder is more common in men?

    a. Borderline
    b. Antisocial
    c. Histrionic
    d. Dependent
    e. All of the above

41) Which of the following is not true of antisocial personality disorder?

    a. It is twice as common in males as in females
    b. It is twice as prevalent in inner cities as in rural areas
    c. Antisocial behaviours do not develop after the age of 18
    d. Spontaneous remission may occur in middle age
    e. It is characterized by excess mortality

42) Regarding psychodynamic theories of aetiology of personality disorders, all of the following are correctly paired, except:

    a. Paranoid personality–Projection of castration anxiety
    b. Histrionic personality–Difficulties at the oedipal stage
    c. Dependent personality–Fixation at the oral stage
    d. Obsessive personality/compulsive personality–Difficulties at the anal stage
    e. Borderline personality–Enduring rage and self-hatred caused by sustained neglect and early traumatic experiences

43) All of the following are requirements for a diagnosis of anorexia nervosa, except:

    a. Body weight below 20% of the normal or expected weight for the age and height
    b. Self-induced weight loss
    c. Body image distortion
    d. Endocrine disorder of the hypothalamo–pituitary–gonadal axis
    e. Amenorrhoea in women and loss of sexual interest and potency in men

44) The physical signs and complications of anorexia include all of the following, except:

    a. Bradycardia
    b. Peripheral oedema
    c. Hypothermia
    d. Mitral valve stenosis
    e. An increase in ventricular:brain ratio on neuroimaging

45) All of the following are common blood abnormalities in anorexia, except:

   a. Hyperkalaemia
   b. Hypophosphataemia
   c. Hypercholesterolaemia
   d. Hypercarotenaemia
   e. Hypomagnaesemia

46) Higher prevalence of anorexia is found in all of the following, except:

   a. Females
   b. Higher socioeconomic class
   c. Patients whose parents have a low level of education
   d. Western Caucasians
   e. Ballet or modelling schools

47) Which of the following is true of bulimia nervosa?

   a. It shares the same specific psychopathology of fear of fatness as anorexia nervosa
   b. It involves recurrent episodes of over-eating at least twice a week for a period of 3 months
   c. It is associated with craving for food
   d. Metabolic acidosis occurs in laxative abuse
   e. All of the above

48) Which of the following statements is false?

   a. The female:male ratio in bulimia is the same as that in anorexia
   b. Average age of onset is slightly lower in bulimia than anorexia
   c. Social class distribution is slightly more even in bulimia than anorexia
   d. Patients with bulimia can be of normal weight, slightly underweight or overweight
   e. In bulimia, menstrual abnormalities occur in more than 50% of patients

49) All of the following statements about Diogenes syndrome are true, except:

   a. It occurs in elderly people
   b. It is characterized by extreme hoarding of rubbish
   c. Alcohol or frontal lobe dysfunction may play a part
   d. Its most common cause is schizophrenia
   e. It is associated with poor prognosis

50) Regarding cross-cultural psychiatry, all of the following statements are true, except:

a. Catatonic schizophrenia is more common in developing countries
b. Hysteria is more common in developing countries
c. Many cultures do not have the language to express the same feeling of depression as described in the West
d. Schizophrenia as defined by operational research criteria is not higher in people of Afro-Caribbean origin living in the UK compared with British White people and Asians
e. Immigrant groups have a higher rate of suicide by burning, with a nine-fold excess among Indian women

12. Clinical psychiatry 5: Answers

1) b.

Kraepelin developed the concept of dementia praecox; Kahlbaum described catatonia.

2) e.

When severe disruption of work and symptoms that lead to social rejection occur, the illness is classified as mania.

3) b.

For the diagnosis of bipolar affective disorder, ICD-10 requires two or more episodes of disturbance in a patient's mood or activity level. These could be either one episode of depression and one episode of mania/hypomania, or two episodes of mania/hypomania. A single episode of mania with psychotic symptoms cannot be classified as bipolar disease.

4) d.

The hallucinations and delusions may or may not be mood congruent.

5) a.

Learned helplessness is the cognitive theory that explains depression.

6) c.

Male first admissions with depression continue to climb until the end of life, overtaking women at the age of 85.

7) e.

Paranoid and delusional ideation, denial of low mood, complaints of loneliness, etc. are common.

8) a.

The Geriatric Depression Scale focuses entirely on cognitive symptoms and is thus helpful.

9) d.

It is characterized by four or more episodes in 12 months; it is more common in women; lithium is relatively ineffective; 20% of cases are triggered by antidepressants.

10) e.

Bipolar I refers to major depression alternating with mania; bipolar II is major depression alternating with hypomania.

11) b.
The lifetime risk of bipolar disorder (BPD) is 1% and of unipolar disorder (UPD) 10–20%; in first-degree relatives of people with BPD, lifetime risk of BPD is 10% and of UPD 2%; in first-degree relatives of people with UPD, lifetime risk of BPD and UPD is 10–15%; the male:female sex ratio for BPD is 1:1 and UPD 1:2; the average age of onset of BPD is 21 years and UPD 27 years.

12) e.
In certain families, manic depressive illness has been X-linked to colour blindness and glucose-6-phosphatase deficiency.

13) e.
83% of patients with Cushing's syndrome develop affective disorder. Hypoparathyroidism is also associated with depression.

14) d.
Suicide is more common in men and people over 45, among those who are single, divorced or widowed, and in social classes I and V. Rates are higher in spring and early summer.

15) b.
50% of psychiatric patients who commit suicide suffer from depression.

16) d.
Deliberate self-harm is more common in lower social classes.

17) a.
The scale awards one point to the following criteria in addition to the other choices given in the question: age above 45; male; not married; poor physical health; psychiatric disorder; and previous suicide attempt.

18) a.
Hecker subdivided neurasthenia and Freud distinguished between actual neuroses and psychoses. Tyrer introduced the general neurotic syndrome.

19) d.
Post-traumatic stress disorder is classified under F43, which deals with severe stress and adjustment disorders; under this, PTSD is classified separately as F43.1 and adjustment disorder as F43.2.

20) c.
About 25% of people exposed to a potentially traumatic event develop post-traumatic stress disorder.

21) b.

The DSM-IV diagnosis of acute stress reaction requires decreased awareness of the surroundings.

22) e.

In ICD-10, grief reaction is classified under 'Adjustment disorders', F43.2.

23) b.

Social phobias are equal in both sexes.

24) e.

Anxiety symptoms are not secondary to other symptoms such as delusions or obsessional thoughts.

25) e.

Familial aggregation and a three-fold elevated risk of social phobia in relatives have been identified, but no specific chromosomes have been identified.

26) d.

Most cases begin in the early or mid-20s, and there is a further period of high onset in the mid-30s. Simple phobias begin in childhood and social phobias in the late teens or early 20s.

27) e.

Panic disorder requires unpredictable attacks of severe anxiety lasting usually for a few minutes only.

28) d.

Stressful life events are more associated with late-onset generalized anxiety disorder.

29) d.

Obsessive compulsive disorder is rare in children, there is an equal sex ratio, patients perform poorly on shifting set, and the prognosis in males with early onset is poor.

30) d.

Favourable prognostic factors in obsessive compulsive disorder also include short duration of symptoms, whereas males with early onset, need for symmetry and exactness, the presence of hopelessness, hallucinations or delusions, and family history of OCD are associated with poor prognosis.

31) e.
Dissociative or conversion disorders are associated with traumatic events, insoluble problems or disturbed relationships.

32) e.
Malingering is feigning illness with an obvious motivation.

33) c.
Dissociative amnesia is more common in young adults and is rare in elderly people; memory loss caused by organic states and fatigue is excluded; recovery is complete and recurrence is unusual.

34) c.
Dissociative fugue is precipitated by severe stress; it is characterized by amnesia for the period of stress, though self-care and social relationships are preserved.

35) d.
Pseudohallucinations are a principal feature of Ganser syndrome.

36) e.
Only one personality is evident at a time and one personality does not have access to memories of the other. Couvade's syndrome occurs in men whose partners are pregnant; symptoms include morning sickness, abdominal pain and anxiety.

37) e.
Somatization disorder is characterized in ICD-10 by 2 years of symptoms. It begins before the age of 30. It was described by the St Louis group and named after Briquet, who wrote a monograph on hysteria.

38) e.
The separate validity of body dysmorphic disorder has not yet been established and there are overlaps with delusional disorder, hypochondriasis and obsessive compulsive disorder.

39) a.
Schizotypal personality disorder is included in DSM-IV.

40) b.
Antisocial personality disorder is described in DSM-IV. Features include: callous, transient relationships; irresponsible, impulsive and irritable behaviour; lack of guilt and remorse; and failure to accept responsibility.

41) a.
The male:female sex ratio in antisocial personality disorder is 7:1.

42) a.
One of the characteristics of paranoid personality is projection of homosexual impulses.

43) a.
Body weight below 15% is needed for a diagnosis of anorexia nervosa.

44) d.
Mitral valve prolapse occurs in anorexia.

45) a.
Hypokalaemia is a common blood abnormality in anorexia.

46) c.
Higher prevalence of anorexia is found in patients whose parents have a higher level of education.

47) e.
High prevalence of depression, self-mutilation, attempted suicide, substance abuse and low self-esteem are seen in bulimia.

48) b.
Average age of onset is higher in bulimia than anorexia.

49) d.
Diogenes syndrome is mostly unaccompanied by any psychiatric disorder.

50) d.
Schizophrenia as defined by operational research criteria is higher in people of Afro-Caribbean origin living in the UK compared with British White people and Asians.

Further reading

Gelder M, Harrison P, Cowen P. *Shorter Oxford Textbook of Psychiatry*, 5th edn. Oxford: Oxford University Press, 2006.

ICD-10: *The ICD-10 Classification of Mental and Behavioural Disorders: Clinical Descriptions and Diagnostic Guidelines*. Geneva: World Health Organization, 1990.

Puri B, Hall A. *Revision Notes in Psychiatry*, 2nd edn. London: Arnold/ Hodder Education, 2004.

Sadock BJ, Sadock VA. *Kaplan and Sadock's Synopsis of Psychiatry*, 10th edn. Baltimore, MD: Lippincott Williams and Wilkins, 2008.